ARTHRITIS

How to Stay Active and Relieve Your Pain

*Barbara Stokes and
Antoine Helewa*

BULL PUBLISHING COMPANY
BOULDER, COLORADO

Arthritis: How to Stay Active and Relieve Your Pain

Copyright © 2007 Bull Publishing Company

Bull Publishing Company
P.O. Box 1377
Boulder, Colorado 80306
(800) 676-2 55   Fax (303) 545-6354
www.bullpub.com

ISBN: 978-1-933503-03-5

Manufactured in the United States of America

Publisher: James Bull
Editor: Erin Mulligan
Production/Interior Design: Dianne Nelson, Shadow Canyon Graphics
Illustrations: Publication Services
Index: Emily Sewell

Library of Congress Cataloging-in-Publication Data

Stokes, Barbara.
    Arthritis: how to stay active and relieve your pain / by
Barbara Stokes and Antoine Helewa.
        p. cm.
    Includes bibliographical references and index.
    ISBN 1-933503-03-3
    1. Arthritis—Popular works. I. Helewa, Antoine. II. Title.
RC933.S785 2007
616.7'22—dc22
                                    2007036516

3755 0612 5/08

Contents

*This book is dedicated to our families and to the
many people we have known who live with arthritis
and from whom we have learned so much.*

Barbara Stokes and Antoine Helewa

Preface

Writing a self-help book for individuals with arthritis is a challenging endeavor. When we decided to write this book, we knew that many other books had been written covering one aspect or another of arthritis care. But we felt there was still no single comprehensive book that focused on the incredibly complex variety of physical and psychosocial problems facing arthritis sufferers while also presenting scientifically sound, practical advice that would provide a measure of relief from these problems. So we set out to write a book with a simple goal in mind—to help people address the daily challenges that individuals with arthritis face and offer them solutions that are *achievable* and *self-directed* and that can result in a vastly improved quality of life.

In addition to its comprehensive coverage of a wide range of simple and practical treatment choices, our book is unique in that it presents the scientific evidence to support these treatments. In recent years we have seen a marked growth in all fields of arthritis research resulting in scientifically-proven fresh approaches to disease assessment, diagnosis, and treatment. In this book we do our best to explain, in everyday language, what these scientific achievements are and how they can benefit individuals with arthritis. We believe that presenting the scientific basis for treatment options equips people to make the best informed choices about their own arthritis care.

What We Cover

The word "arthritis" has become a generic term covering the 100 different forms of disease that primarily affect joints and their related structures. Many of these distinct disease entities share common symptoms and methods of treatment. Because of this, we focus on those diseases that are most common and share symptoms and treatment approaches rather than cover each disease entity separately. For example, *rheumatoid arthritis,* a common and debilitating form of arthritis, shares characteristics and treatment approaches with *juvenile chronic arthritis, psoriatic arthritis* and *systemic lupus erythematosis.* Since the similarities among some diseases are greater than the disparities, we have grouped related forms of arthritis together. We hope that this will make the book equally useful to people with a wide array of diagnoses.

Our Organization

This book is divided into two parts. Part 1 explains what arthritis is, discusses its impact on the individual (and society); describes how human joints do their job; lists the common forms of arthritis; and provides information about community resources for individuals with arthritis. Other chapters in Part 1 cover scientific research (and how it informs treatment choices); detail the importance of arthritis medications in controlling the disease process; and address the issues of arthritis pain management, wellness, and disability prevention with a special emphasis on the great importance of physical exercise in arthritis treatment.

Part 2 of the book offers specific advice on how individuals can self-manage their arthritis. The first three chapters cover exercise, building on the foundation established in Part 1. The benefits of different types of exercise are discussed and simple exercise guidelines are provided and illustrated. Exercises that increase joint mobility, improve muscle strength and endurance, and boost aerobic capacity are key components of any program and are covered here in detail. Part 2 also explains how to protect joints from damage and conserve energy; how to adjust to the emotional and social impact of arthritis; how to enjoy happy and healthy intimate relationships; and how to make good lifestyle choices. The two final chapters of the book cover arthritis surgery options and explore the claims of some alternative arthritis treatments. An appendix lists even more resources and organizations which exist to support individuals as they cope with their arthritis.

Scientific researchers in the treatment of arthritis have made great strides in the last decade and the support resources for people with arthritis are also expanding with every passing day. The future is brighter than ever as we continue to learn more about how people with arthritis can stay active and control pain. Our goal in this book is to help you make sense of all the valuable information that is available. Our deepest hope is that our book will help *you* to take control of *your* arthritis and live the full and rewarding life you deserve.

Acknowledgments

We are grateful to Gail Paterson, BScPT, The Arthritis Society, Ottawa, Canada, and Maureen Czop, a Patient Partner™, Perth, Ontario, Canada, for their assistance in preparation of the illustrations of self examination in Chapter 2. Maureen acted as the model and Gail shot the photographs from which the drawings were produced.

Our thanks go to Jim Bull, Publisher; Erin Mulligan, Editor; Dianne Nelson, Shadow Canyon Graphics; and Publication Services for the support, encouragement, and skill that made our vision of this book a reality.

Foreword

For patients with arthritis, this is a most welcomed publication on how to manage their problem, written by two knowledgeable and experienced physical therapists who have both practiced and taught extensively in the field. The authors have produced a comprehensive, easy-to-read, and understandable book on arthritis in terms of what it is, how it may impact on the patient, and its management. Although the focus is primarily on self-management, important areas such as diagnosis, the role of various health professionals, medications, and surgical options are also dealt with.

This is essentially a book on "all you want to know about arthritis" and "important advice about arthritis which doctors and other health professionals may not tell you." Apart from important factual information, the book is also interesting reading for patients in terms of the historical aspects of the disease and the structure and function of joints. Particularly useful are the sections on diagnosis, the assessment of disease activity and extent of joint involvement, and how to seek appropriate help. In this day and age when so much material is available from a vast number of sources, advice provided by the authors on how to sort out what is appropriate, potentially effective, and not harmful, based on sound scientific evidence is very relevant.

This book, written by experts in the area is a "must read" and important source of useful information for all patients who are afflicted with arthritis and other causes of joint pain. While it is important to listen to the advice of health professionals involved in the treatment of arthritis, it is also important for the patient to know what they can do to help themselves. This book provides appropriate information on how this can be accomplished.

Dr. Peter Lee, MB, CHB, MD, FRCPC, FRACP
Professor of Medicine
University of Toronto
Rheumatologist
Mt. Sinai Hospital
Toronto, Ontario, Canada

List of Abbreviations

AS	Ankylosing Spondylitis
BMI	Body Mass Index
BRM	Biologic Response Modifiers
CAHC	Complementary and Alternative Health Care
DMARD	Disease Modifying Antirheumatic Drug
ECG	Electrocardiogram
FM	Fibromyalgia
GLA	Gamma-linolenic acid
JCA	Juvenile Chronic Arthritis
MD	Doctor of Medicine
MSW	Master of Social Work
NCCAM	National Center for Complementary and Alternative Medicine
NSAID	Non-steroidal Anti-inflammatory Drug
OA	Osteoarthritis
OT	Occupational therapist
OTC	Over-the-counter
PsA	Psoriatic Arthritis
PhD	Doctor of Philosphy
PT	Physical Therapist
RA	Rheumatoid Arthritis
ROM	Range of Motion
SLE	Systemic Lupus Erythematosis
TENS	Transcutaneous Electrical Nerve Stimulation
TGV	Thunder God Vine
WHO	World Health Organization

Part 1

Finding Out About Arthritis

Chapter 1

What Is Arthritis and What Can I Expect from This Book?

This book is for people who suffer from arthritis and diseases closely related to arthritis. It addresses the general effects of this group of diseases as well as issues relating to drug and surgical management. While providing the reader with a broad overview of the disease, the book primarily focuses on the self-management of arthritis:

✦ How to stay mobile and flexible with physical exercise.

✦ How to cope with and relieve pain using simple at-home methods.

✦ How to protect joints and conserve energy during daily activities.

✦ How to deal with the emotional and social effects of arthritis.

✦ How to make healthy lifestyle choices.

✦ How to assess the potential for harm or benefit from both traditional and non-traditional remedies.

Chapter 1 explains what arthritis is, the history of the disease and its treatment, and the cost it incurs on society. Once these basics have been covered, the chapters that follow focus on various disease-management issues for people with arthritis. This book is divided into two parts. Part I, Finding Out About Arthritis, provides the basic background information you will need as you make decisions about managing your arthritis. Part II, Getting Healthy and Staying Well, gives you practical advice and useful tools to live a healthy and productive life with arthritis.

ARTHRITIS AND ITS SYMPTOMS

The term "arthritis" is derived from *arthro*, the Greek word for a joint, and *itis*, the Latin word for inflammation. It is used to describe more than 100 different disorders of joints and the structures that surround them, such as ligaments, tendons, and muscles. These conditions share a common feature: inflammation. If inflammation is left untreated, it can lead to changes within the joints and in the tissues that surround them. These changes cause pain, stiffness, deformity, and difficulty in performing normal activities of everyday life. Arthritis has long been associated with old age and severe deformities, but in reality, it is not age-dependent. It affects children and adults of all ages.

Arthritis can be mild and localized to a single joint, tendon, or bursa (a fluid-filled sac that reduces friction among moving parts); or it can be severe, affecting most of the joints in the body as well as major body systems. Arthritis due to wear and tear is often referred to as osteoarthritis, or OA. This degenerative form of arthritis can affect all moving joints. OA is seen in the elderly and in those whose joints have been subjected to repeated injuries. It is by far the most common form of arthritis, and it affects both large and small joints. It causes pain and deformities and, in severe cases, can lead to artificial joint replacement.

For people with OA and other milder forms of arthritis, premature death is not a factor, but pain and disability can increase with age, reducing the quality of life. Severe forms of arthritis, referred to as "systemic" (such as rheumatoid arthritis [RA], lupus, juvenile arthritis, and ankylosing spondylitis [AS]), affect joints, muscles, arteries, the heart, the lungs, the kidneys, the intestines, and the skin with various degrees of severity. RA begins with joint swelling and inflammation and can affect small and large joints that produce movements. In severe cases, it can affect all body systems. RA and the systemic forms of arthritis can lead to early death as a result of the disease, or due to its complications and treatments. However, in spite of these potentially serious complications, very few people with systemic forms of arthritis in the western world are currently severely disabled or immobilized by the disease.

There are more than 100 different types of arthritis, and joint inflammation is common to all.

Early symptoms of most forms of arthritis include pain, swelling, stiffness in joints, fatigue, stress, depression, and sleeping problems. Unless it is treated, the disease can lead to the destruction of joint structures and difficulties in performing normal activities.

In addition to physical symptoms, stress and depression are common among people with arthritis. Stressors are life events with which an individual cannot cope and that are seen as threats to well-being. Stressors associated with arthritis include the challenges of coping with a long-term chronic health problem, restricted activities, uncertainty about the future, long-term disabilities, and direct and indirect economic losses. These stressors may contribute, in turn, to psychological distress that poses additional threats to physical and emotional well-being.

The depression most often seen in people with severe forms of arthritis is a mixture of anxiety and depression. It increases the perception of pain and is influenced by pain. Loss of the ability to perform valued activities can be a leading cause of depression. Studies show that even after their depression has been successfully treated, people with a history of depression who have rheumatoid arthritis are vulnerable to higher levels of pain, fatigue, and disability.

A large number of people with arthritis in the northern hemisphere say that their symptoms of pain are worse in colder months such as December and January, and are least severe in July. However, these perceptions are not supported by X-ray and laboratory measures taken by clinicians. One reason for this may be that changes in atmospheric pressure affect joint structures and increase the perception of pain. Another factor may be that the depression that can accompany bad weather heightens the sense of suffering in some people.

HISTORY OF ARTHRITIS

Arthritis has been discovered in human and animal fossils dating back more than one million years. More recent evidence of arthritis has been seen in the joints of Neanderthal remains, in excavated mummies of ancient Egyptian royals, and in skeletal remains from the Roman and Saxon periods. In the eighteenth century, the bony thickenings near the tip of the fingers seen in the hands of the elderly were first described and distinguished from the nodes or outgrowths found in patients with gout. These arthritic outgrowths, or "Heberden's nodes," were named after the physician who first described them and are depicted in paintings and sculptures dating to the fourteenth century A.D. These nodes are typical of OA of the finger joints. In contrast to OA, evidence of RA has not been found in old skeletons. This suggests that RA, one of the most severe forms of arthritis, may be of recent origin.

It was during World War I and World War II that physicians first took notice of arthritis in army recruits during pre-enlisting medical examinations. Nearly all of these recruits were men, and the type of arthritis that was most prominently noted was the type still typically found in young men today: ankylosing spondylitis, or AS. AS affects the spinal column and related structures and can spread to other large joints such as the hips, the knees, the shoulders, and the elbows. Like RA, it can also affect body systems with the same serious results.

Osteoarthritis has been found in prehistoric human and animal fossils, whereas rheumatoid arthritis is thought to be of more recent origin.

The historical record shows that the physical treatment of arthritis dates back to the third century B.C. The Greeks and Romans valued the use of massage and hot-water immersions to treat arthritis. In eighteenth-century England, moderate exercise such as walking and riding was recommended. In the early twentieth century, Osler, a renowned Canadian-born physician, recommended fresh air, a healthy diet, hot baths, massage, and exercise to improve joint movements. In the western world, between 1910 and 1920, it was believed that arthritis was the result of a bacterial infection. In order to remove suspected sites of infection, vast numbers of teeth, tonsils, gall bladders, and other organs were extracted. Irrigation of the large intestines "to rid the body of toxic wastes" was also a popular form of treatment.

The goals of arthritis treatment are to control pain and inflammation and to prevent disability.

Currently, the mainstays of physical treatment for people with arthritis are:

✦ General exercise—in and out of water—to strengthen muscles, increase joint movements, and promote aerobic fitness.

✦ Lifestyle adaptations.

✦ General patient education.

✦ Simple pain-relieving modalities, such as hot packs or ice packs.

Modern testing methods have made it possible for physicians, other health professionals, and scientists to develop ways to identify, classify, and treat the various forms of arthritis. These efforts led to the creation of rheumatology as a distinct medical specialty and research area in the 1950s.

During that same period, the Arthritis Foundation in the United States, the Arthritis Society in Canada, and other sister organizations throughout the world were formed. These organizations are dedicated to funding arthritis research, providing patient education, and promoting modern treatment methods.

Currently, very few arthritis patients in developed countries are wheelchair-bound or bedridden, largely due to better control of joint inflammation and destruction and continually evolving pharmaceutical, surgical, and physical treatment methods.

ARE WE IN THE MIDST OF AN ARTHRITIS EPIDEMIC?

Population surveys show that about 16 percent of North Americans complain of arthritis symptoms. In 85 percent of those complaining of arthritis symptoms, the duration of the typical episode of arthritis was longer than one year. More women (18.8 percent) than men (13.2 percent) reported these complaints; this is largely due to the longer life span among women and to the fact

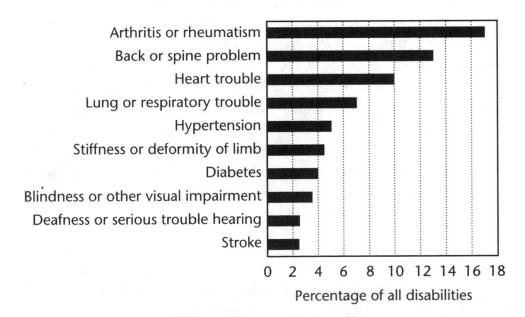

Figure 1-1
Sixteen percent of all North Americans complain of arthritis, a higher number than complain of any other ailments listed in this graph.

that certain common forms of arthritis, such as RA, affect women three times more often than they affect men. In 1981, 55 percent of those sixty-five years and older had arthritis, while among those fifteen to sixty-four years of age, the occurrence was 17 percent. In children fourteen years and younger, only 1.3 percent were affected.

Public perception is that arthritis is seen more often now than in decades past. This is because certain forms of arthritis, such as osteoarthritis, occur most frequently in older people, and since people are now living longer, there are more elderly people alive today suffering from arthritis than there were in the past. In addition, many of the post–World War II baby boomers, who are health-conscious and intent on remaining physically fit, have subjected their joints to frequent and often lifelong traumas by adhering to intensive running, jogging, and exercise regimes. Even when proper footwear and running gear are used, running and jogging can cause shin splints. As these minute bony fractures heal, deposits of hard, unyielding bone replace the original, more resilient, shock-absorbing bone. With repeated injuries, the resiliency of long bones, such as those in the lower legs, is diminished, subjecting the cartilage that lines the joint surfaces to increased stress. This, in turn, causes damage to the cartilage and can lead to the onset of traumatic osteoarthritis (OA caused by repeated injury). As boomers grow older and live longer, they will be increasingly plagued by this wear and tear, adding to the number of patients with arthritis. "

**Moderate jogging can keep you fit and mobile;
excessive running and jogging
can damage your joints.**

And so, while there is no epidemic of arthritis, more people with arthritis are around today due to the increase in life span and changes in modern lifestyles. You will probably continue to hear more about arthritis in the next three decades as these trends continue.

The Price of Arthritis

The impact of arthritis on the lives of individuals and their families can be unsettling. Arthritis limits the ability of more than seven million Americans to work, attend school, and participate in other activities of daily living. By the year 2020, about 12 million Americans will experience significant limitations due to this illness.

The direct costs of arthritis in the United States in 1995 (medical and hospital care, drugs, home adaptations and transportation) amounted to $22 billion, and the indirect costs (lost wages

Table 1-1
Direct and Indirect Costs of All Musculoskeletal Conditions and
All Forms of Arthritis (in billions of 1995 dollars)

Condition	Direct Costs	Indirect Costs	Total Costs
All musculoskeletal conditions	88.7 (41%)	126.3 (59%)	215
All forms of arthritis	21.7% (26%)	60.8 (74%)	82.5

In 1995, the costs of arthritis to the U.S. society and economy exceeded $80 billion. Adapted from Praemer, Furner, and Rice.

due to a reduction or cessation of work) totaled $61 billion. The costs of arthritis extend beyond these direct and indirect costs, however. It is impossible to put a dollar value on the toll it takes on the lives of patients, including pain, disability, stress, disruption of family life, loss of independence, and changes in appearance due to deformity.

Arthritis is the leading cause of work loss and the second leading reason why people receive disability payments. In addition to working, activities that may be difficult or impossible for people with arthritis include using transportation, shopping, housecleaning, cooking, interacting with family and friends, and participating in hobbies. All of these problems have negative effects on society's productivity and on government revenue. Add to these the personal effects of arthritis on the individuals and families who must somehow learn to cope with this chronic condition, and it becomes apparent what an enormous burden arthritis places on society.

In 1995, the costs of arthritis to society and the economy in the United States exceeded $80 billion.

Looking Forward

Society needs new strategies to cope with arthritis and its impact in order to protect the well-being of citizens without bankrupting the health-care system. This book offers important self-help strategies to teach people who have arthritis how to manage the disease in a positive manner. A balanced approach is taken to present treatment options, address pain relief, and teach you how to avoid disability. Promoting self-care and reducing the pressure on the patient and on the health-care system are its principal goals. Better public information, self-management of joint inflammation, and focused and appropriate exercise will reduce the burden of arthritis on individuals and on society as a whole. It is hoped that you will learn valuable information that will give you options for leading a healthy and pleasurable lifestyle with arthritis.

The next chapter includes a description of joints and the effects of joint inflammation and degeneration on joint structures, as well as a self-assessment guide to help determine which joints are affected by this disease. The remaining chapters in the first part of this book address the physical, emotional, and psychological effects of arthritis. The second part of the book features concrete, usable advice on how to cope with these challenges.

Chapter 2

What Are Joints and How Do They Work?

It is important that people with arthritis understand the physical composition of joints (structure) and how the joints work (function) in order to comprehend the disease process and control its effects on physical activities. Chapter 2 begins by providing a general outline of the structure and function of the joints responsible for moving the limbs and trunk. These joints are called synovial joints, due to the presence of the thick, slippery, synovial fluid. The chapter then briefly discusses the way in which arthritis can damage joint structures, the specific features of certain key synovial joints, and the way in which joint disease may interfere with normal joint function. At the end of the chapter, you will find a joint-by-joint self-assessment of joint inflammation.

WHAT ARE SYNOVIAL JOINTS AND HOW DO THEY MOVE?

Synovial joints feature a lubricant referred to as synovial fluid, which reduces friction between joint surfaces during movement. This fluid is not present in other types of joints. Synovial joints are freely movable. The shoulders, elbows, and knees are examples of synovial joints, whereas the joints connecting the vertebral bodies in the spine, and the joints that connect the bones of the skull, are not.

Your freely movable joints are synovial joints.

In a typical synovial joint (Figure 2.1):

✦ The bone ends that form a joint are covered with gristle and held together by ligaments.

✦ The gristle covers the bony surfaces in order to reduce friction as the bones move against each other.

✦ The ligaments consist of an inner capsule that contains the synovial fluid and an outer layer of tough tissues that reinforce the capsule.

✦ A membrane lines the capsule and produces the highly slippery synovial fluid, which acts as a lubricant.

✦ Muscles and tendons provide further stability to the joint and supply the power to move it.

✦ Fluid-filled sacs (bursae) lie between the tendon and the bone to reduce friction when these structures move over each other.

✦ Blood vessels are embedded in the joint to provide nutrition to the joint structures.

✦ Nerves are also embedded in the joint. Nerves register pain sensations and provide a sense of direction as the joint moves.

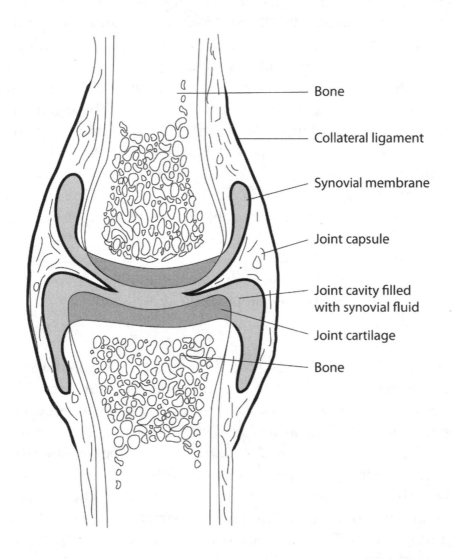

Bone

Collateral ligament

Synovial membrane

Joint capsule

Joint cavity filled with synovial fluid

Joint cartilage

Bone

Figure 2.1
Synovial joints are freely movable and contain synovial fluid.

How Many Types of Synovial Joints Are There?

Synovial joints differ according to their line (or axis) of movement. Uniaxial or hinge joints allow movement along one axis (up and down or side to side).   To get an idea of how these joints work, imagine a door hinge. The elbows, knees, ankles, and joints of the fingers and toes are examples of uniaxial joints—their "hinge" structure allows them to bend or stretch.

Ellipsoidal and saddle joints are biaxial synovial joints that allow movement along two axes (*axes* is the plural of axis). These joints are often shaped like an ellipse. The wrists, knuckles, and joint at the base of the thumb are examples of biaxial joints; they allow for bending and stretching as well as for sideways movement. You can see the knuckle joints in action when you open your hand and spread your fingers to hold a large object, such as a grapefruit.

**The three types of synovial joints
each move in different ways.**

The third type of synovial joint is referred to as a ball-and-socket joint and is multiaxial. The hip and shoulder joints are examples of ball-and-socket joints. They allow the joint to bend and stretch, move sideways (as in spreading the legs), and rotate (roll outward or inward). Figures 2.2, 2.3, and 2.4 illustrate the three types of synovial joints and the ways in which they move.

This characterization of synovial joints is a simplified description that does not take into account mathematical complexities of joint movements. Of course, joints do not move in isolation but are part of body processes that allow several joints to move in a pattern. For example, serving a ball in tennis involves movements

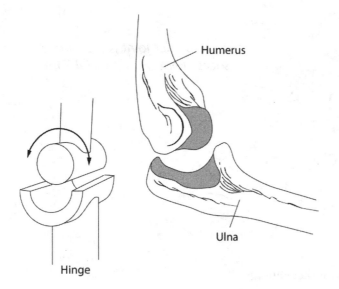

Humerus

Ulna

Hinge

Figure 2.2
The elbow joint is an example of a hinge or uniaxial joint; it moves in only one direction.

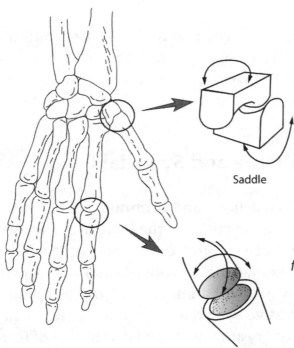

Saddle

Ellipsoidal

Figure 2.3
The knuckles are ellipsoidal or biaxial joints; they move forward and back as well as from side to side

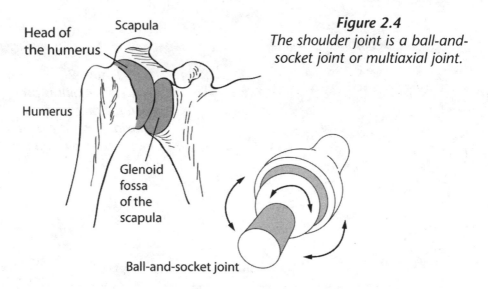

Head of the humerus

Scapula

Humerus

Glenoid fossa of the scapula

Ball-and-socket joint

Figure 2.4
The shoulder joint is a ball-and-socket joint or multiaxial joint.

of fingers, wrists, elbows, shoulders, the head, the neck, and the trunk and lower limbs. This complex of movements produces a multiaxial pattern aimed at delivering an exact and powerful serve of the tennis ball to your opponent.

The Synovial Membrane and Synovial Fluid

The synovial membrane is a delicate and continuous sheet of tissues rich in blood vessels. It covers all of the structures enclosed within the joint capsule but does not cover the cartilage. The membrane produces a clear and sticky synovial fluid with a consistency much like egg whites. Inflammation of the membrane (synovitis) produces excessive synovial fluid that is less sticky than the fluid produced by a healthy joint and therefore is of inferior quality. Laboratory tests of the fluid can be a valuable aid to diagnosis.

Healthy synovial fluid is necessary for healthy joints.

The fluid plays an important part in joint lubrication and nourishment of the joint cartilage. In healthy joints, it reduces the amount of friction on joint surfaces during movement and makes the joint surfaces more slippery than ice sliding on ice. This is beneficial because the body utilizes the replaceable fluid to reduce friction rather than the irreplaceable joint surface. Under normal circumstances, there is only a small amount of fluid present in a joint, but when the synovial membrane is attacked by disease, a large quantity may be produced, causing a stretching of the joint capsule and swelling of the joint. This excess fluid is typically less sticky, which reduces its lubricating quality. Uncontrolled inflammation and the presence of poor-quality synovial fluid can eventually cause destruction of joint structures. Synovial fluid, a great asset for normal joint function, becomes a liability in joint disease.

The Role of Cartilage

Adult cartilage or gristle lining the joint surfaces receives its nourishment from the synovial membrane and small blood vessels embedded in the joint capsule and underlying bone. There are no sensory nerves embedded in cartilage; therefore, it does not convey pain sensations or position sense. Cartilage is resilient and elastic and acts as a shock absorber during normal movements and weight bearing. Due to the special arrangement of its fibers, its surface is very smooth. In this way, it aids in reducing friction when surfaces glide over each other. By the time we reach adulthood, our cartilage has lost most of its ability to grow and repair itself.

Cartilage cushions our joints.

Despite continuous use, there is no evidence that cartilage cells are worn away in healthy joints. However, if joint disease is present or trauma such as fractures inside the joint occur, the cartilage will degenerate and quickly wear away. When the cartilage disappears from the joint surfaces, the "cushion" is lost, and bone rubs directly on bone. A joint without enough cartilage has a reduced ability to withstand shocks. This phenomenon is common in diseased joints, and this is why arthritis treatment is aimed at protecting affected joints from further cartilage reduction.

The Role of the Joint Capsule, Ligaments, and Associated Structures

The joint capsule with its reinforcing ligaments is responsible for containing the synovial fluid within the joint cavity, as well as for holding the joint together (see Figure 2.1). Capsule fibers are several millimeters thick and are reinforced by ligaments. These ligaments may be found outside of the capsule and may be situated inside or outside the joint. The capsule and ligaments provide strength but very little elasticity. During joint movement, the capsule tends to fold into accordion-like folds on one part of the joint while it becomes taut on the opposite side. This arrangement of fibers restrains undesirable movements. For example, in the knee joint, taut ligaments on either side restrain side-to-side movements as you bend and stretch the joint. They also hinder movement when the knee is fully bent or fully stretched to prevent overstretching. When you have arthritis, joint inflammation can lead to stretching of the joint capsule and joint deformity, or "looseness" or laxity. This condition may be aggravated by excessive movement or weight bearing.

WHY IS JOINT MOVEMENT IMPORTANT?

For people with arthritis, moving an inflamed joint can be painful. In that case, a protective mechanism kicks in that informs muscles not to act on such a joint. Take the case of a joint that is inflamed with excessive low-quality synovial fluid in the joint cavity. This excess fluid puts a strain on the joint capsule and ligaments, producing pain. Certain joint angles allow the joint to accommodate more excess fluid than other positions. For example, an inflamed knee joint may be painful when it is fully stretched or fully bent, because the joint holds the least amount of fluid in these positions. If that same knee is slightly bent, it holds more fluid, reducing the stress on the capsule and ligaments and therefore reducing the amount of pain. Thus, a person with arthritis in the knee may naturally hold the knee in a slightly bent position. In time, the structures around the joint adapt to this limited angle, reducing the joint's ability to move freely. Reduced joint movement results in muscle weakness and reduced joint function.

WHAT DETERMINES IF A JOINT IS INFLAMED?

The most common joint complaints among arthritis patients include swelling or enlargement around a joint, tenderness to pressure, and/or stress pain at the end of the joint's range of motion. Other symptoms include heat, redness, and loss of movement (Table 2.1).

Table 2.1
Symptoms of Joint Inflammation

Common Patient Complaints When Joints Are Inflamed

Pain
Stiffness
Deformity
Loss of function
General malaise

What a Health-Care Provider Is Looking for in a Joint Examination

Heat
Redness
Swelling
Loss of movement
Deformity
Tenderness
Abnormal movement
Crackling sounds
Inability to perform normal activities

Joint inflammation can result in pain, stiffness, and swelling, among other symptoms.

Swelling

Swelling or enlargement around a joint can be due to excessive synovial fluid inside the joint. This is often referred to as an effusion. Swelling or enlargement can also be due to inflammation of related tissues outside the joint, enlargements and distortions in the shape of bones forming a joint, or the presence of fat pads around a joint. It is important that a health-care provider determine which of these is the cause of the enlargement and whether the enlargement is due to bony changes or effusion.

Effusion appears as a palpable bulging of the joint. If compressed, the fluid will shift and add to the distention of the joint elsewhere. The fluid thus fluctuates within the joint. A normal joint contains just enough synovial fluid to act as a lubricant, and this small quantity of fluid is not palpable—that is, it cannot normally be felt under the examiner's fingers or manipulated. The presence of palpable fluid in a joint is an indication that the joint is inflamed. As mentioned earlier, to avoid the discomfort resulting from excessive fluid in a joint, people tend to hold an affected joint in the position where it most comfortably accommodates the greatest amount of fluid. For example, an effused knee joint will be slightly bent, an ankle will be pointing downward, and an elbow will be slightly bent. Attempts to stretch or bend these joints further will result in pain when they are swollen.

Joint effusions are commonly found in the inflammatory forms of arthritis such as rheumatoid arthritis. Inflamed joints are not usually seen in patients with osteoarthritis; the visible joint enlargement seen in OA tends to be bony and not due to inflammation of the synovial membrane (synovitis). In bony enlargements, the bony surfaces of a joint look distorted and out of shape.

Tenderness

In affected joints, the tissues close to the joint line (the place where the two ends of a joint come in contact) tend to get inflamed. These areas can be very tender to touch due to the underlying inflammation. When this inflammation is present, finger pressure at the joint line will result in pain. Joints where effusion is not palpable, but are tender to pressure near the joint line, are considered inflamed. This is commonly the case with inflamed uniaxial joints, such as the knees and finger joints.

Stress Pain

A normal joint that is taken to the limit of its movement and then a little bit past will produce a sensation of stretching. An inflamed joint, if taken to the limit of its movement and then a little bit past, will be very painful. This is referred to as stress pain. This occurs because the inflamed synovial membrane is stretched at the end of the range of motion. For a joint to be labeled as inflamed, pain must be felt within the joint itself, not in muscles or tissue close to the joint. The experience of stress pain is another indicator of joint inflammation.

A joint is inflamed when:
There is an effusion.
There is tenderness at the joint line.
Pain is experienced at the extremes of movement.

ARE MY JOINTS INFLAMED?

Determining whether or not individual joints are inflamed or effused is a difficult task and an art form in its own right. This task is usually left to physicians, physical therapists, and occupational therapists with special training in rheumatology. However, in the following section, we provide guidelines to determine if your joints are inflamed. This self-assessment will help you to judge the extent and severity of your arthritis. Of course, it is always necessary to have any joint-inflammation assessment or arthritis diagnosis confirmed by a medical professional.

In joint examination, the presence of any effusion, tenderness to pressure, or stress pain is a sign of underlying joint inflammation. Of these three indicators, an effusion is the most reliable sign of joint inflammation. To determine the extent of a person's arthritis, a joint map is used to identify the most common inflamed joints. (See Figure 3.2 in the next chapter for an example of a joint map.) When the number of affected joints is tallied, this list forms an index. As you might expect, a person with thirty-five inflamed joints is much worse off than a person with five inflamed joints.

Identifying Inflammation in Key Joints

A person with arthritis can learn to identify inflamed joints through self-examination techniques that are similar to those used by health-care professionals. Some joints, seen in Figures 2.5–2.14, are easier to score than others and are therefore selected for that purpose. The following tips can help you to identify and measure the presence of joint inflammation by monitoring tenderness or stress pain. Checking for effusion or swelling is more complex and is best left to the professionals. If you find that your joints are inflamed, contact your physician to learn more about the extent and cause of the inflammation.

Joints of the Jaw

Place the tips of your index and middle fingers on either side of the joint line just in front of the opening to your ear (Figure 2.5). Apply pressure with the tips of your fingers at the joint line and feel for tenderness; or open and close your mouth, which will put stress on the joint.

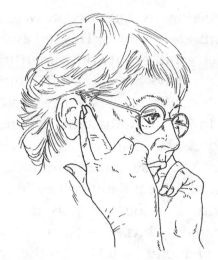

Figure 2.5
Checking for inflammation in the joints of the jaw.

Shoulder Joints

With your elbow bent, hold your arm away from your body and rotate your shoulder while maintaining the arm and elbow position (Figure 2.6). When the shoulder is rotated as far as possible, apply pressure on your forearm and check for pain in the joint.

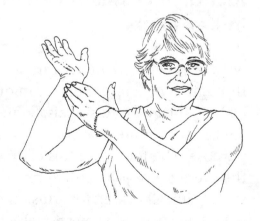

Figure 2.6
Checking for inflammation in the shoulder joints.

Elbow Joints

Place your fingers over the grooves at the back of your elbow and apply pressure to feel for tenderness (Figure 2.7).

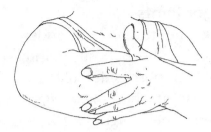

Figure 2.7
Checking for inflammation in the elbow joints.

Wrist Joints

Bend your wrist forward as far as possible and apply pressure over the back of your hand to check for tenderness in the joint (Figure 2.8).

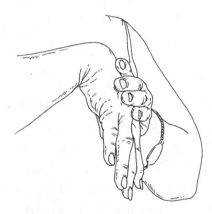

Figure 2.8
Checking for inflammation in the wrist joints.

Knuckle Joints

With the opposite hand, extend the five knuckle joints one at a time for signs of stress pain (Figure 2.9).

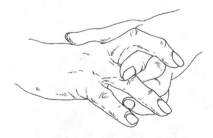

Figure 2.9
Checking for inflammation in the knuckle joints.

Finger Joints

With the thumb and index finger of the opposite hand, press on both sides of each finger joint, checking for signs of tenderness (Figure 2.10).

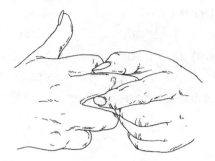

Figure 2.10
Checking for inflammation in the finger joints.

Hip Joints

To test for stress pain, sit on a chair with your feet resting on the floor. Slide your feet away from each other, but keep your knees together (Figure 2.11). If the joint is inflamed, pain will be felt in the groin.

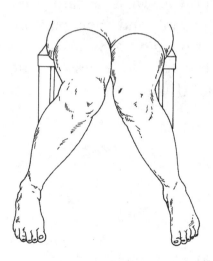

Figure 2.11
Checking for inflammation in the hip joints.

Knee Joints

To test for tenderness, sit on a chair with your feet resting on the floor, and apply pressure with the fingertips of both hands to the inside and outside of the knee at the joint line (Figure 2.12).

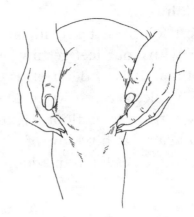

Figure 2.12
Checking for inflammation in the knee joints.

Ankle Joints

Sit on a chair with your feet resting on the floor, then raise your toes slightly. Press your foot straight down against the floor without moving any other part of the your body (Figure 2.13). Pain within the ankle joint will indicate inflammation.

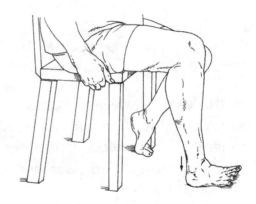

Figure 2.13
Checking for inflammation in the ankle joints.

Toe Joints

To test for stress pain, sit on a
chair with your feet resting on
the floor. Raise one heel at a
time while keeping your toes
pressed against the floor (Figure
2.14). Pain within any of the
joints indicates inflammation.

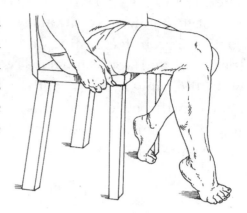

Figure 2.14
Checking for inflammation in
the toe joints.

Looking Forward

In this chapter, we covered the essential anatomy and function of
synovial joints. We also discussed how individual joints become
inflamed and provided guidelines to help you assess your joints so
that you can gain an awareness of the extent and seriousness of
your arthritis.

Chapter 3 introduces you to the most common and serious
forms of arthritis by describing their symptoms and their effects
on body systems. It also tells you about important tests that are
useful to diagnose each form of arthritis and assess its severity.

Chapter 3

Is Arthritis One Disease or Several?

While joint inflammation and degeneration are the main symptoms of arthritis, these characteristics coexist with a variety of symptoms that can be mild or severe. They may be localized, or they may affect nearly every system in the human body. At last count, scientists and specialists working in this field had identified more than 100 distinct conditions that come under the label of arthritis and rheumatism. Of these, the majority are rare, with strange-sounding names such as Behçet's disease (also known as Silk Road disease because it is most prevalent in countries along the old Silk Road) or Marfan's syndrome (which manifests itself in excessive bony growths and abnormal body proportions). Although their names may be unique and varied, many of the inflammatory types of arthritis have similar or overlapping symptoms, and most are treated with similar types of drugs and therapies.

The first section of this chapter serves as a guide to detecting key symptoms of arthritis and includes a brief description of their management. It is followed by detailed content about the most common forms of arthritis and their origin, symptoms, and treatments. This chapter lists and describes only the most common joint disorders and their symptoms. These include inflammatory joint diseases such as rheumatoid arthritis (RA), systemic lupus erythematosis (SLE), juvenile chronic arthritis (JCA), ankylosing spondylitis (AS), psoriatic arthritis (PsA), reactive arthritis, scleroderma, and gout. The order of presentation of the inflammatory arthritis types in Chapter 3 takes into account the incidence and the severity of these diseases. Also covered in this chapter is the degenerative joint disease best known as osteoarthritis and the diffuse pain condition known as fibromyalgia. Table 3.1 lists the common types of arthritis and rheumatic diseases. We do not cover conditions that are localized to specific areas, such as bursitis, tendonitis, and carpal tunnel syndrome, although they often coexist with the disorders listed above.

DETECTING AND MANAGING COMMON ARTHRITIS SYMPTOMS

Figure 3.1 (page 36) is a flow chart that will help you to identify symptoms and determine steps to take if your pain and discomfort are the result of arthritis. The first box describes "red flags"—serious health problems (that may or may not be related to arthritis) for which you must seek immediate medical help. Subsequent boxes tell you how to proceed if your primary complaints are related to one or more joints, or if they are due to generalized muscle pain. By proceeding down the chart, you can distinguish between forms of arthritis that start with joint inflammation (such as

Table 3.1
Classification of the Common Forms of Arthritis

INFLAMMATORY JOINT DISEASES

    Rheumatoid arthritis (RA)

    Systemic lupus erythematosis (SLE)

    Juvenile chronic arthritis (JCA)

    Ankylosing spondylitis (AS)

    Psoriatic arthritis (PsA)

    Reactive arthritis

    Scleroderma

    Gout

DEGENERATIVE JOINT DISEASES

    Osteoarthritis (OA)

DIFFUSE PAIN SYNDROMES

    Fibromyalgia (FM)

rheumatoid arthritis), forms of arthritis that are due to gout or joint infection, arthritis associated with psoriasis, or arthritis associated with degeneration or "wear and tear" (such as osteoarthritis).

Consult your family or primary-care physician first before you seek treatment from anyone else.

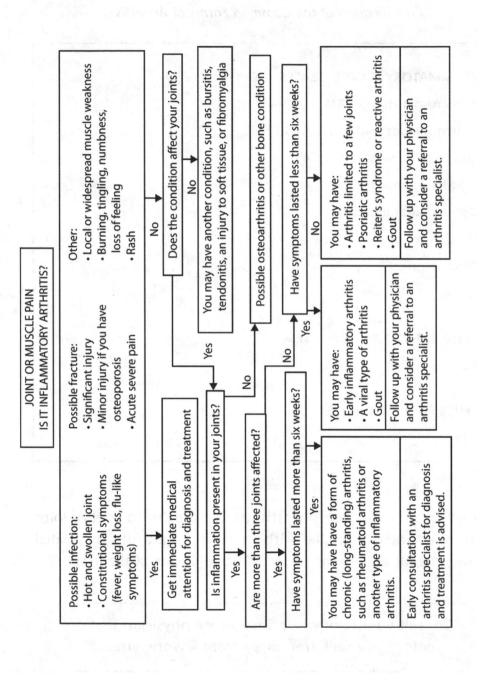

Figure 3.1

Is your joint or muscle pain a sign of inflammatory arthritis?

At various points in the flow chart, you are advised to seek the help of your family or primary-care physician. Make sure that any physician you see has a medical degree and a license to practice medicine. His or her name should be followed by the letters "MD," indicating that he or she is a medical doctor or physician. Not all those who are referred to with the title of "doctor" are MDs. Some are doctors of philosophy (PhDs), while others may be chiropractors, osteopaths, podiatrists, or naturopaths.

We advise you to visit your family physician (not a chiropractor, osteopath, or naturopath) first—for two reasons. First, your family physician carries the *pass key* to the rest of the health-care system. If you need access to other specialists or treatments, your primary-care physician is the best contact to help you locate and utilize these services. In many managed-care situations, you can only see a specialist once your primary-care physician has referred you. Second, primary-care physicians are trained to identify and screen problems related to *all* systems of the human body. This is important, especially if you have inflammatory arthritis, which often affects several body systems.

If you are unable to reach the physician who treats your arthritis, your arthritis is severe, and you are running a temperature, go to the closest emergency department at a hospital.

Your family physician may decide to personally treat your arthritis if it is mild, or he or she may refer you to an arthritis specialist or rheumatologist if your case is moderate or severe. If there is no access to a rheumatologist in your community, your primary-care physician may decide to refer you to a specialist in internal medicine. If your condition requires surgery, your doctor may refer you to an orthopedic specialist. If your condition requires physical rehabilitation, you may be referred to a physical or occupational therapist. Chapter 4 covers this topic in more detail. Always remember that, if you are unable to reach the physician who treats your arthritis, your arthritis is severe, and you are running a temperature, go to the closest hospital emergency department as soon as possible.

ARRIVING AT AN ACCURATE DIAGNOSIS

The first task of your family physician or specialist is to interview you to create a complete detailed medical history of your current episode, your past illnesses, and those of your immediate family members. A physician will listen to your current complaints, such as pain, stiffness, sweats, fever, fatigue, and loss of function. He or she will ask you to list all of the medications you currently take, your dosages, and any side effects. The interview process will be followed by a general physical examination of your system of joints and muscles (musculoskeletal system).

In cases of inflammatory arthritis, such as rheumatoid arthritis, your physician will determine the number of joints involved (Figure 3.2). In addition, he or she will screen for problems in other body systems and organs. These include the heart and blood vessels (the cardiovascular system), the lungs and bronchi (the respiratory system), the stomach and intestines (the gastrointestinal system), the kidneys, the liver, the skin, the nervous system, the urinary tract, and the genitalia. Your doctor may also order blood and urine tests, as well as X-rays of any affected joints.

The examination will generally also include questions about your living and work environments. You should share information about any limitations the symptoms are imposing on your

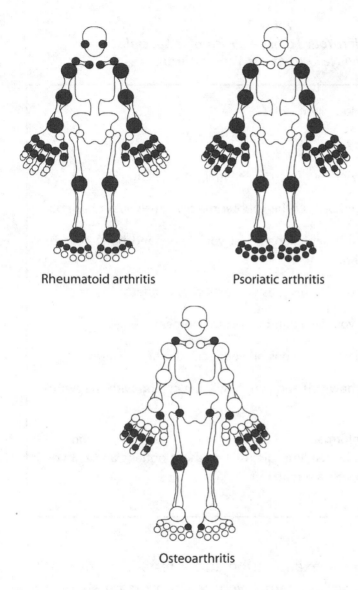

Rheumatoid arthritis   Psoriatic arthritis

Osteoarthritis

Figure 3.2
The circles in this diagram indicate the typical distribution of joints affected in RA, PsA, and OA patients. The higher the joint count, the more severe the disease.

activities of daily living, how you and your family are coping with the symptoms, and any difficulties you may be having when it comes to performing your work responsibilities. Table 3.2 on the next page summarizes the steps your family physician or specialist will take to arrive at a diagnosis of arthritis.

Table 3.2
Information Your Family Physician or Specialist
Will Need to Assess Your Arthritis

1. Your current chief complaint.

2. Your medical history.

3. The medical history of your immediate family, if relevant.

4. A list of all prescribed or over-the-counter medications you are taking.

5. A complete physical examination of all your joints and body systems affected by the arthritis.

6. Results of blood and urine tests, as well as X-rays of affected joints.

7. Information about your living and work environments.

8. Information about any limitations on your activities of daily living.

9. Information about how you and your family are coping with the symptoms of arthritis.

When all the above information is collected and processed, your primary-care physician should be ready to discuss treatment options and tell you whether specialist referrals are required.

After completing the examination and interview, your family physician or specialist may tentatively reach a diagnosis of one or more of the types of arthritis described in the following section. In the early stages of your condition, do not be surprised if your doctor is unable to offer you a definite diagnosis, because many factors need to be looked into before an accurate diagnosis is made.

INFLAMMATORY JOINT DISEASES

The conditions covered in this section all result in joint inflammation. They share common symptoms and treatments, with minor differences. The order in which they are presented takes into account disease severity and incidence. We begin with the most common form of inflammatory arthritis, rheumatoid arthritis (RA).

Rheumatoid Arthritis (RA)

RA is a chronic disease of unknown cause that results in inflammation of one or more synovial joints. About 1 percent of the total adult population is affected—three times as many women as men have the disease. People on every continent are at risk of getting RA, but the disease tends to be less common in Asia and Africa.

A diagnosis of RA depends greatly on the medical history and physical examination and less on standard laboratory tests. While early diagnosis is important in order to start early treatment, a definitive diagnosis is not always easy to confirm.

In RA, the joints affected tend to be symmetrical. This means that the disease similarly affects corresponding joints on both the right and left sides of the body. It usually starts with joint swelling (synovitis) and pain associated with joint use, accompanied by morning stiffness and loss of movement in the joints. This stiffness, which is most noticeable upon waking, can last from fifteen minutes to four hours depending on the severity of the RA. For most people, this stiffness gradually lessens so that they can resume normal activities as the day progresses.

RA usually starts by affecting the small finger and toe joints. The disease can then progress to the larger joints, such as the ankles, knees, hips, wrists, elbows, shoulders, jaw, and spine. RA symptoms can result in loss of physical function, interruption of sleep, stress, and reduced quality of life.

An early diagnosis of arthritis improves your chances of controlling joint destruction.

Flu-like symptoms are common—perspiration, a slight elevation of body temperature, and weight loss. In addition to affecting the musculoskeletal system, RA may also seriously affect other organ systems, including the cardiovascular, respiratory, and nervous systems. In women, the presence of certain sex hormones may play a role in the activity of RA. Pregnant women sometimes experience relief from symptoms due to increased production of cortisone during gestation. However, the period after birth, when there are decreased levels of natural cortisone in the system, can be challenging, as the symptoms may return with a vengeance.

The progression of RA is quite variable. If the disease is left untreated, joint damage and physical disability will likely develop. The disease usually lasts a lifetime; very few patients experience complete relief of symptoms.

The cause of RA remains unknown. Various theories have been advanced. Some of these theories have focused on genetic factors, because RA tends to run in families, and identical twins share a diagnosis more often than fraternal twins. Other factors associated with the disease include low income levels, low education levels, high stress levels, environmental risk factors, and prior exposure to infections (viral or bacterial). A recent research study in Sweden suggested that some or all of the above factors may combine to reduce the body's defense mechanisms, leaving individuals vulnerable to RA.

Because the effects of RA on the individual can be significant, early aggressive treatment is needed. The goals of treatment are outlined in Table 3.3.

Table 3.3
The Goals of Treatment for Rheumatoid Arthritis

---

1. Patient education.

2. Control of joint inflammation.

3. Pain control.

4. Restoration of joint function.

5. Joint protection and energy conservation.

6. Surgical correction of destroyed joints.

7. Emotional and social support.

Patient Education

Once the diagnosis of RA is made, you can accomplish the first goal of RA treatment by asking your family physician for information in the form of self-help books or brochures from the Arthritis Foundation in the United States, The Arthritis Society in Canada, or other sister associations across the world. If you have access to the Internet, you can access web sites for these organizations, which provide well-balanced, up-to-date perspectives on the disease and its management. Please see the resources section at the end of this book for more information on patient-education resources.

Control of Joint Inflammation

In the early stages of RA, it is extremely important to reduce joint inflammation and the destructive effects it can have on joint tissues (see Chapter 2). A large number of drugs are available to control inflammation:non-steroidal, anti-inflammatory drugs (NSAIDs); disease-modifying, anti-rheumatic drugs (DMARDs) (disease-modifying drugs are typically drugs that suppress the immune system); cytotoxic agents, such as corticosteroids and methotrexate, which also suppress the immune system; and a new group of drugs called biologic agents, which reduce the inflammatory process that leads to joint destruction. Corticosteroid injections inside the joint may also be prescribed if joints do not respond to oral medications. Please refer to Chapter 6 for more detailed information about these drugs, their uses, and their possible side effects.

Pain Management

You can control your pain using standard pain medication, or natural pain-relieving strategies such as cold packs or hot packs. The drugs mentioned in the previous paragraphs also help control pain by controlling inflammation. Please refer to Chapter 7 for further information about pain-management techniques.

Restoration of Joint Function

Strong scientific evidence indicates that exercise in its various forms is the ideal way to maintain and restore joint function. Three forms of exercise are recommended: exercise that keeps joints moving, also called range-of-motion exercise; exercise that strengthens or maintains muscle strength; and aerobic exercise (in or out of the water), which helps to increase or maintain endurance for normal activities. Exercise does not need to be excessive. Taking a walk is an excellent way to get exercise. If your feet, ankles, or knees are affected by arthritis, you may need a walking aid or shoe inserts to avoid putting undue stress on your lower joints. These types of exercises are usually taught by a physical therapist. Please refer to Chapters 9, 10, 11, and 12 for more details about the best types of exercises to engage in to get and stay strong, mobile, and fit.

Joint Protection and Energy Conservation

RA can have a destructive effect on joints; therefore, once it is diagnosed, you will want to find ways to protect your joints. You will also need to learn how to carry out your daily activities in a way that helps you to conserve your energy, since RA affects all systems of the human body and causes fatigue. You can learn special ways to do things that can help you get the most out of your daily energy expenditure and the most mileage out of your joints. These special techniques are often called joint-protection and energy-conservation techniques and are usually taught by occupational therapists. Please refer to Chapter 13 for more details on these techniques.

Pacing activities and protecting joints will help you to reduce fatigue and preserve your joints.

Surgery

Surgical correction of destroyed joints and related tissues is used as a last resort. Surgeries include partial or complete replacement of joint surfaces by artificial materials (arthroplasty); surgical bonding of joint surfaces (arthrodesis); repair of frayed tendons or ligaments; and surgeries to relieve pressure on trapped nerve tissues. For more information about surgical options and techniques, please see Chapter 17.

Support

Because RA is a chronic disease, it usually lasts a lifetime. Psychological and emotional distress related to the disease is common in arthritis patients. The emotional impact of the disease is usually addressed by psychologists or medical social workers. More serious psychiatric problems may require a referral to a psychiatrist. Other forms of social assistance are also sometimes needed to help patients cope with the extra expenses resulting from the disease and its treatment.

It is important to note that treatment of RA requires a coordinated effort by a health-care team, with each member of the team assuming responsibility for one or more of the goals listed above. At the center of this team effort is *you*, the patient. You have a responsibility to report difficulties and to carry out personal health-management tasks negotiated with other team members. More details on the roles and functions of health-care team members are available in Chapter 4.

Systemic Lupus Erythematosis (SLE)

Also known simply as lupus, SLE is one of the most serious forms of arthritis. It specifically targets blood vessels, the heart, the lungs, the kidneys, the nervous system, and the skin, as well as muscles and joints. Lupus alternates between periods where the disease is more active, called exacerbations or flare-ups, and periods where there is little or no inflammation, called remissions.

In lupus, as with RA, the immune system that normally protects the body from germs and bacteria begins to malfunction. It generates cells, called antibodies, that attack healthy tissue in various parts of the body, causing inflammation. Lupus is eight to ten times more common in women of childbearing age (ages fifteen to forty-five) and occurs less frequently in men and children.

Lupus is a different disease for each person it affects, because it can involve any of the body's tissues; each person suffers from his or her own combination of symptoms. Lupus usually manifests with a combination of the following symptoms:

✦ Pain in the muscles and swelling in the joints, accompanied by red, hot, and swollen skin.

✦ Fatigue, fever, loss of appetite, and frequent, severe headaches.

✦ Painless sores in the mouth and nose.

✦ Sensitivity to sunlight.

✦ Skin rashes, frequently seen across the cheeks and bridge of the nose as a "butterfly rash," and often seen in a less severe form of lupus.

✦ Chest pain, high blood pressure, and swelling of the feet.

✦ Sudden changes in body weight.

It might take a period of time before a diagnosis of lupus is made, because the symptoms differ from person to person. If your family physician suspects that you have lupus, a referral to a rheumatologist is very important. After thoroughly considering the combination of symptoms and test results, and after ruling out other conditions, a rheumatologist may confirm a diagnosis of lupus. However, there is no single symptom, sign, or test that can confirm a definitive diagnosis of lupus.

The cause of lupus is unknown, but family members of lupus patients may be affected with the disease as well, indicating that the disease may have a genetic component.

The whole range of drugs prescribed for RA is often indicated for lupus patients as well. The aim of drug treatments is to bring lupus symptoms under control and bring about a remission of the disease. Early drug management can reduce the effects of the disease on body tissues, thereby averting permanent damage to affected organs. This can also lessen the amount of time an individual with lupus needs to stay on high doses of medications.

Physical exercise to increase joint mobility, muscle strength, and endurance is essential to controlling the symptoms of lupus and reducing flare-ups of the disease. Physical exercise can also help allay stress. If you are diagnosed with lupus and plan to exercise outdoors, use sunscreen, as too much exposure to sunlight can trigger a flare-up. Employing joint-protection techniques to reduce stress on inflamed joints and making use of tips on how to save energy while performing physical tasks can lessen the symptoms of fatigue.

Most people with an early diagnosis of lupus who receive early treatment can look forward to a normal lifespan, in spite of periodic disease flare-ups. The majority of people with lupus do not require hospitalization or intensive treatment and can lead a normal life.

Juvenile Chronic Arthritis (JCA)

Arthritis in children, also known as juvenile chronic arthritis, or JCA, is a group of systemic inflammatory joint diseases affecting children younger than sixteen years of age. In the United States, roughly 100 out of every 100,000 children are affected by JCA. Although JCA is much less common than RA, it is a major cause of disability in childhood. Overall, more girls are affected than boys, and JCA can strike at any age during childhood. Some affected children develop stunted growth of their long bones; others experience overgrowth of these same bones. Either of these conditions can lead to one limb being shorter or longer relative to the other.

Three major types of arthritis are found in children: pauciarticular, polyarticular, and systemic onset.

Pauciarticular JCA

In this type of JCA, four or fewer joints are involved; it is found in 60 percent of children with JCA. It is more common in girls than boys and affects children before the age of five. Pauciarticular arthritis strikes at the knee most often; the ankle joint is the second most affected joint. This may lead to a noticeable limp but very little pain. Seventy-four percent of girls in this group also have eye disease (uveitis) that must be monitored by an ophthalmologist every three months. Eye disease occurs in conjunction with the other forms of JCA as well, but less frequently.

Polyarticular JCA

In polyarticular JCA, five or more joints are involved; it is found in 30 percent of children with JCA. It is most common in girls twelve to sixteen years of age. It may affect all the small joints of the hands and feet and is equally distributed on both sides of the body (symmetrical). Like RA, it can also affect body systems. The prognosis (how the disease progresses and ends) is less favorable for polyarticular JCA than it is for the pauciarticular form.

Systemic-Onset JCA

Systemic-onset JCA strikes about 10 percent of children with arthritis. It may start with a high, spiking fever, a salmon-pink rash over the upper parts of the body and extremities that comes and goes, and joint problems. It can affect abdominal organs, the heart, and the lymph nodes, and it may cause enlargement of the liver and the spleen. Fifty percent of affected children recover completely, especially if a limited number of joints is involved. In the remaining 50 percent of patients, the disease progresses, resulting in varying degrees of physical disability.

Children with JCA often go into remission and outgrow the disease by adolescence, but early treatment is still critical to prevent joint stiffness and uneven bone growth that can result in serious disabilities.

How Is JCA Treated?

Treatment goals for JCA follow the same pattern as those listed for RA in Table 3.2. Education of the child and family about the disease and its long-term effects is very important. To prevent isolation of affected children, information about JCA should be made available for schoolteachers, coaches, and other caregivers.

Families, teachers, and coaches must be educated about the disease so that they can effectively assist children with JCA to participate fully in normal daily activities.

Medications to control inflammation must be safe and simple to monitor and administer. Most patients start with high doses of NSAIDs (and sometimes coated aspirin), in conjunction with physical-therapy measures to control pain and restore normal joint movement. The joints of these children can become stiff very quickly, and exercise to mobilize the joints is essential in the early stages of JCA. Swimming and other water exercise keeps joints mobile and muscles strong. Corrective splints are usually needed to hold the joints in a normal functional position when the child is at rest or sleeping.

If the disease continues to progress, then other medications may be prescribed, such as low doses of DMARDs, or, in very extreme cases, low doses of oral corticosteroids. Corticosteroid injections inside the joint may also be needed if one or two joints are not responding to oral medications. More recently, drugs such as etaneracept have been used in severe cases. You can read more about drugs used to treat arthritis in Chapter 6.

Counseling of the child and family by social workers is important for normal family functioning and to address the guilt that parents of these children often report feeling. It is vital to the child's development that he or she be kept active and engaged socially and academically. To ensure normal childhood development, it is important that affected children not miss out on the fun of being a child. Teachers must be brought into the "fold" and educated about the condition and the particular needs of the patient.

Please refer to Chapters 9, 10, 11, and 12 for more details about mobilizing, strengthening, and endurance exercises that are recommended for the treatment of JCA.

Ankylosing Spondylitis (AS)

Ankylosing spondylitis, or AS, is a chronic disease that results in inflammation, pain, and stiffness in all the joints of the spinal column and, to a lesser extent, the larger joints of the arms and legs. It is part of a group of arthritic diseases that are linked together by a genetic factor (HLA-B27) and other common symptoms. These include psoriatic arthritis, Reiter's syndrome (a rare disease that causes arthritis, inflammation of the urinary tract, and inflammation of the membrane that lines the eyelids), and arthritis associated with inflammation of the bowels. AS is common in Caucasians (one to two per thousand), and Haida Indians (four per thousand), but is rare among the Japanese, Australian aborigines, and Native Africans. It is most common in men between the ages of fifteen and forty-five. The spinal pain of AS is often mistaken for common low-back pain; therefore, the prevalance of the disease is difficult to determine.

AS is common among male Haida Indians and Caucasians between the ages fifteen and forty-five.

AS usually first strikes at the joints that connect the pelvis to the lower spine (the sacroiliac joints) and gradually spreads up the spine. The inflammation begins at the point where tendons attach to bones (enthesis) and can cause either loss of bone cells (resorption) or new bone formation (ossification). The bony changes caused by AS fuse the vertebral bodies of the spine together and obliterate the joint spaces of the spine that normally are seen on X-rays. The affected joint spaces include the facet joints, which link the arches of the vertebrae together; the intervertebral discs, which link the vertebral bodies together; and the joints that link the ribs to the spinal column. Because these bony changes make the spine on an X-ray look like a bamboo stick, this phenomenon is often referred to as "bamboo spine."

The end result of the progression of the disease is a rigid spine and a limited ability to move the trunk, along with a rigid rib cage, which limits chest expansion and causes breathing difficulties. A major problem for individuals with AS is the development of a severe and permanent bending or flexion of the spine. If this deformity is allowed to progress, walking becomes difficult due to poor balance, and maintaining an upright posture while sitting, standing, or propped up in bed is challenging. Those who are severely affected and allow their symptoms to go untreated tend to walk with a rounded back and a jutting chin. Because they have difficulty raising their head, they tend to roll their eyeballs upward to be able to see what is ahead. This form of arthritis may also affect the hips, knees, shoulder joints, and heels in a similar manner.

The general symptoms of AS are:

✦ Low-back pain that may spread down the buttocks and thighs. As the disease progresses, the pain and stiffness move up the spine.

✦ Spinal stiffness that is worse during periods of rest and improves with exercise.

✦ Limited movement in the lower spine.

✦ Stiffness of the rib cage and reduced chest expansion, which make breathing difficult.

✦ Pain and stiffness in the shoulders, hips, knees, and the heel area.

✦ Loss of the normal curves of the spine, a rounded back, and a poking chin.

✦ Eye symptoms, such as iritis or inflammation of the iris.

✦ In severe cases, there is narrowing of the spinal canal, which results in pressure on the spinal cord and causes weakness of muscles and tingling and loss of skin sensation.

AS treatment has similar goals to those of RA but also distinct differences because of the body parts that are affected and the greater prevalence of AS among young men. Treatment goals for AS are outlined in Table 3.4. Overall, the similarities in the treatment of AS and RA are greater than the differences.

Table 3.4
The Goals of Treatment for Ankylosing Spondylitis

1. Patient education.

2. Control of joint inflammation.

3. Pain control.

4. Maintenance of correct posture during walking, standing, sitting, and sleeping positions.

5. Maintenance of rib-cage mobility and lung function.

6. Maintenance and restoration of movement of the spinal column and extremity joints.

7. Joint protection and energy conservation.

8. Career counseling.

9. Emotional and social support.

Education

Education about the disease for the individual, his or her family, employers, friends, and coworkers is very important in order to increase understanding of the disease process and facilitate coping with its effects on daily functioning. Career counseling for those affected, who tend to be mostly men in the prime of life and often primary providers for their families, is of great assistance.

Medication to Control Joint Inflammation

As is the case with RA, NSAIDs are commonly used to control joint inflammation for AS patients. DMARDs such as methotrexate can control this form of arthritis in the extremities, but these drugs are ineffective in the treatment of the spine. Short courses of oral corticosteroids also help control the inflammation in badly affected extremity joints. Iritis requires referral to an ophthalmologist or eye specialist and is usually treated with corticosteroid eyedrops.

Pain Control

The treatment of joint pain and stiffness is similar to the treatment for pain in RA patients.

Maintenance of Posture and Mobility

Maintaining mobility of the spine through range-of-movement exercises is very important for AS patients. However, as the disease progresses, this becomes a difficult task. The maintenance of an upright posture is one important aspect of treatment. If spinal movements begin to become limited, the patient must do exercises to correct posture using mirror feedback. Postures during walking, standing, sitting, and lying in bed should be corrected. If the spine becomes rigid, it should be maintained in an upright rather than a rounded position.

Postural exercises may reduce the incidence of rounded backs and poking chins for people with AS.

Maintenance of Rib-Cage Mobility

Rib-cage rigidity can be reduced with deep breathing exercises to maintain rib-cage and lung expansion. Limited chest movement reduces the individual's endurance for physical activities and increases the risk of respiratory diseases.

**Exercise is the cornerstone
of AS management.**

Joint Protection and Energy Conservation

Joint-protection and energy-conservation techniques reduce stress on affected joints and improve performance of physical activities.

Career Counseling

Career counseling by members of the treatment team, especially occupational therapists and social workers, is an important part of disease management for AS patients who are active in the workplace. Such counseling helps to maintain work performance by modifying the workplace to accommodate patient needs. Counseling can also help individuals deal with the emotional, psychological, and social effects of the disease. Interestingly, AS patients tend to deal very well with their limitations, and they maintain a more positive view of life than other individuals with chronic arthritis.

Psoriatic Arthritis (PsA)

Psoriasis is a relatively common condition in which scaly red and white patches develop on the skin. Between 5 and 7 percent of patients with widespread psoriasis will develop the form of arthritis referred to as psoriatic arthritis, or PsA. In the United States, one tenth of 1 percent (0.1 percent) of the population is affected by this disease. It most often affects young and middle-aged adults, and it affects men and women equally. The exact causes of psoriasis and psoriatic arthritis (PsA) are not known, but they are both thought to be due to environmental or genetic factors, since 40 percent of patients with PsA have a family history of psoriasis. Like RA, PsA results when the body's autoimmune system, which normally exists to protect against invading organisms, goes into overdrive and causes excessive inflammation. Like psoriasis, PsA can cause symptoms that periodically show up (flare) and then subside. Fifty percent of patients have changes in their nails that may consist of nail pitting and nail-plate crumbling. Fatigue and anemia are common, and some patients have mood changes.

In some people, PsA is mild and comes and goes; in other people, it can cause persistent symptoms that lead to joint damage if not treated.

The pattern of joint involvement can vary. In some individuals, PsA affects the joints near the tips of the fingers (joints that are usually not affected by RA). Another form can cause severe destruction or mutilation of the joints of the hands (and occasionally the feet) and shortening of the fingers or toes. A third form resembles RA clinically with a similar distribution of joint involvement. A fourth form may involve one to a few joints and result in a dactylitis (a sausage-looking finger or toe). A fifth form tends to affect the spine, mimicking ankylosing spondylitis (see the previous section in this chapter for more information about AS). Both psoriasis and psoriatic arthritis tend to get worse in the winter months when patients typically get less exposure to sunlight.

The treatment goals for PsA are similar to those of RA (see Table 3.3). However, patients with PsA do not have to continually take medications; instead, they need doses only when symptoms arise.

Skin lesions caused by PsA may require special attention and are often treated with artificial ultraviolet rays, preceded by the application of special skin creams (emollients) consisting of petroleum products (petrolatum) or other creams such as psoralen.

Reactive Arthritis

Reactive arthritis results from a previous infection; it causes swelling, pain, and stiffness in affected joints. It affects mostly the knees, ankles, and toes, and, rarely, the upper limbs. In some patients, it can also involve other parts of the body, such as the eyes, skin, muscles, or tendons. When this is the case, it is referred to as Reiter's syndrome.

Patients with reactive arthritis may experience the following symptoms:

+ Pain and swelling in the lower limb joints that appear for no particular reason a few weeks following food poisoning or the contraction of a sexually transmitted infection.

+ Pain in the lower back, heels, or bottoms of the feet.

+ Pain and stiffness that is worse on waking up.

+ Eyes that are sore and sensitive to sunlight.

+ Mouth and genital sores that may or may not be painful.

+ Anemia or reduction in the number of red blood cells resulting in paleness, weakness, sleepiness, or dizziness.

+ In women, irritation of the cervix.

+ Urinary tract infections (urethritis) in both men and women.

Reactive arthritis affects men and women between the ages of twenty and fifty who may experience a bout of food poisoning or be afflicted with some other bacterial infection, such as shigella, salmonella, campylobacter, or yersinia. It also affects those with an inherited genetic tissue: the HLA-B27. This tissue is found in 6 to 10 percent of Caucasians, and its presence is thought to increase the risk of developing reactive arthritis after a sexually transmitted bacterial infection, such as chlamydia or gonorrhea. Fifty percent of patients with reactive arthritis have a positive HLA-B27.

Reactive arthritis is not contagious or sexually transmitted from person to person. Sometimes reactive arthritis goes away on its own in a matter of days or weeks; at other times, it can take four months or more for the symptoms to disappear. If your family physician suspects a diagnosis of reactive arthritis, he or she will probably refer you to a rheumatologist. A standard history of your illness will be taken, and you will be asked questions about recent travel, illnesses, and infections. There is usually a lag time of two weeks between the infection that triggers the arthritis and the appearance of joint symptoms.

The primary objective of treatment for reactive arthritis is to eliminate the infection that has caused the arthritis and to manage the pain and inflammation. The bacterial infection is treated with antibiotics; if the infection was sexually transmitted, the partner should also be treated. Non-steroidal, anti-inflammatory drugs (NSAIDs) are used to treat the pain and inflammation in the joints. Occasionally, a cortisone injection in an affected joint that is resistant to oral medications can reduce symptoms. If the infection lasts longer than four months, then disease-modifying, anti-rheumatic drugs (DMARDs) may be prescribed.

Hot or cold packs or even a hot shower first thing in the morning can reduce pain and get you going for the day if you have reactive arthritis. Exercise to increase muscle strength around affected joints and improve joint mobility is important. Low-impact aerobics can increase endurance and lessen the symptoms of fatigue. Aids and adaptations to protect joints and energy-conservation skills may also help lessen symptoms.

Scleroderma

Scleroderma, a Greek term meaning "hard skin," is also known as progressive systemic sclerosis. It may also be referred to as systemic sclerosis, since not all forms are progressive (worsen over time). When scleroderma is present, the body's immune system stops working properly and attacks healthy tissue. What causes this reaction remains a mystery. The most obvious sign of scleroderma is the buildup of tough, scar-like, fibrous tissue in the skin. A less obvious change includes damage to the cells lining the walls of small blood vessels (arterioles) that, in turn, causes damage to major organs. Scleroderma is a rare condition affecting five to ten persons per million in all populations studied; it is five times more common in women and appears between the ages of thirty and fifty.

Symptoms of scleroderma include:

✦ The appearance of hard, round or oval, white patches on the skin encircled by a reddish area. The patches are usually seen on the chest, stomach, face, arms, or legs. Small red spots may also appear on the skin.

✦ In another form, a line of thickened skin may appear on the forehead, arms, or legs.

✦ Small, white, chalky lumps may appear under the skin of the fingers. If they break through the skin, they will discharge chalky white ooze.

✦ The skin covering the fingers may become shiny and coarse and may feel woody and dry.

✦ Fingers and toes may become sensitive to cold, turning numb and blue.

✦ Heartburn or problems swallowing.

✦ High blood pressure, if the kidneys are affected.

✦ Shortness of breath, coughing, chest pains, and heartbeat irregularities.

✦ Dry eyes, dry mouth, and, in women, dryness of the vagina.

✦ Pain and stiffness in the joints due to inflammation and tightness of the skin.

There is no single test that confirms the presence of scleroderma, making diagnosis difficult. The best indicators are the skin conditions in the symptoms list described above.

Because there is no cure for scleroderma, treatment is focused on symptom control. NSAIDs such as Naprosyn or high-dose, coated aspirin are the first line of treatment. In severe cases, oral prednisone, or DMARDs such as methotrexate, may be prescribed to reduce inflammation and control the immune system. Patients with skin that is sensitive to cold may be prescribed medications that relax the walls of the small blood vessels of the fingers and toes. Those with kidney problems and high blood pressure may need medications to limit the risk of strokes. Antacids may control heartburn.

Skin care is very important. Creams and lotions such as lanolin cream, baby oil, or cocoa butter work well to keep the skin moist. Baby oil in bathwater can also help, but avoid any soaps that contain perfumes or chemicals. Hands and feet must be kept warm with gloves and socks in cold weather. People with scleroderma must avoid pressure on areas with calcium deposits; if the skin breaks, open sores can become infected.

If you have scleroderma, avoid tobacco use, as it causes the blood vessels to shrink in size. Chew food slowly and many times if you have trouble swallowing, and drink fluids frequently if your mouth is dry. Eating smaller and frequent meals will prevent too much acid from coming up from your stomach and causing heartburn. Artificial tears help keep eyes moist. Exercise strengthens muscles and keeps joints and surrounding skin supple. Aerobic exercise in or out of water will increase endurance. Avoid excess stress on your joints by using aids and adaptations, and conserve your energy by pacing your activities, alternating between heavy and light duties, and taking frequent rests.

The severity of scleroderma varies among individuals. Those with major organ involvement (such as the esophagus, kidneys, or lungs) tend to have more severe disease symptoms. Those with skin involvement only do better in the long term.

Gout

Gout is a form of arthritis caused by the accumulation of uric acid in the body. Uric acid is a waste product that is normally flushed by the kidneys and excreted in the urine. When it is not flushed from the body, it forms crystals that are deposited in the joints and give rise to inflammation, causing redness, swelling, and severe tenderness. The joint of the big toe is most often affected, but gout can also attack other limb joints. Uric acid crystals can be deposited in other areas, such as under the skin, under other soft tissues, in the kidneys, and in the urinary tract. Over time, the attacks may become more frequent, and the uric acid crystals deposited in the joints and surrounding soft tissues can cause destructive changes and ongoing inflammation.

Several factors can trigger an attack of gout. These include consumption of alcohol and certain foods, medications that prevent uric acid from being flushed by the kidneys, and events such as strokes, heart attacks, or surgery. Many people with gout have a family history of the disease.

Men are four times more likely to have gout than women. It tends to affect one in thirty individuals and is more common in countries that enjoy a high standard of living. Fifty percent of people with gout are likely to have more than one attack per year. In past centuries, it was referred to as the "disease of kings," because many royals tended to suffer from gout due to their consumption of alcohol and "rich" foods.

Symptoms of gout include:

✦ Awakening at night due to intense, searing pain in the joints of the big toe, heel, or ankle.

✦ Hot, red, swollen skin and pressure around affected joints.

✦ Hot, red, swollen soft tissues such as muscles and tendons near affected joints.

Physicians need three pieces of information to conclusively diagnose gout: a description of the onset of symptoms; an examination of affected joints; and measurements of uric acid levels in the blood and urine or from a sample of joint fluid. If uric acid levels are high, and associated symptoms are present, then the most likely diagnosis is gout.

During an acute attack of gout, the treatment goals are to control joint inflammation, prevent further attacks and damage to the joints, and prevent the formation of kidney stones. Early diagnosis and treatment can minimize damage to the tissues. NSAIDs usually form the first line of defense in an acute attack. The most commonly used is Indocid, but other NSAIDs, such as Naprosyn, Orudis, and Voltaren, work equally well. If NSAIDs do not control the inflammation, then oral cortisone or cortisone injected into the affected joint will usually work, although oral cortisone is rarely prescribed. Colchicine is also very effective, but due to its side effects, it is also not commonly used.

Hot packs are applied to relax muscles and cold packs can reduce joint pain and soreness. Once the acute attack has subsided, the patient should exercise to strengthen muscles, mobilize joints, and increase endurance.

If your body is overproducing uric acid, your physician will provide you with dietary guidelines, as certain foods and beverages must be avoided. Products that can lead to overproduction of uric acid are caffeinated beverages, alcohol, seafood, and organ meats such as liver and kidneys.

When the acute attack has subsided, treatment of the underlying cause must begin. The disease may be brought about by two causes—an overproduction of uric acid in the body or an inability to eliminate uric acid. Those who overproduce uric acid are treated with allopurinol, while those who are unable to eliminate it are treated with probenecid.

DEGENERATIVE JOINT DISEASE

The term "degenerative joint disease" refers to arthritis caused by "wear and tear" on joints. In Chapter 1, we discussed the potential harm that can be caused by repetitive stress being placed on the joints; degenerative joint disease is the result of that sort of stress.

Osteoarthritis (OA)

Osteoarthritis, or OA, is the most common form of arthritis and an important cause of long-term physical disabilities. It is the prevalent arthritis associated with degeneration. Sixty percent of individuals develop OA before the age of sixty-five, and 20 percent before the age of forty-five. The incidence increases as people age, and by age seventy-five, almost everyone has some changes in at least one joint that are typical of OA. Men and women are equally affected before age forty-five, but after age forty-five, it is more common in women. OA has been linked to certain occupations, such as coal mining, and to injuries incurred during certain sports such as football, tennis, or ice hockey. Athletes who continue to engage in these sports following joint injuries will most likely develop OA within five years. Excessive overuse of joints can also cause OA. Running or jogging does not always cause OA of hips or knees, provided there is no previous injury to these joints due to running on unyielding surfaces, or running in unsupportive shoes.

OA is a slowly progressive deterioration or degeneration. First, the cartilage lining the joint surfaces deteriorates; this is followed by the thickening of the underlying bone. Two types of OA are recognized—primary OA and secondary OA. In primary OA, there is no obvious underlying cause; however, it has been linked to systemic (factors related to body systems), genetic, or environmental factors. There are many causes for the changes seen in secondary OA, including:

✦ Joint inflammation such as that seen in RA.

✦ Joint infection.

✦ Fractures inside the joint, disrupting joint surfaces.

✦ Overuse of joints.

✦ Limbs that are not properly aligned, such as bowed legs or knock-knees.

✦ Unequal leg length.

✦ Being overweight, causing excessive stress on knees and hips.

OA affects mostly the joints of the hands and feet, the spine (both neck and back), and the hips and knees. The number of joints involved can vary. OA tends to affect the same body joints on the right and left sides of the body (bilateral). Individuals with three or more involved groups of joints are considered to have generalized OA. Bony enlargement is common, causing pain on pressure (tenderness) at the joint line. These enlargements can be seen easily in the joints near the fingertips and are often referred to as Heberden's nodes or Bouchard's nodes—named after the physicians who first described them.

When a person has OA, the joints lose their normal shape and can appear enlarged or twisted in unusual positions. Loss of joint movement is related to a type of bony outgrowth called an osteophyte, which can be felt near the joint margins. Erosion of the cartilage lining the joint surfaces results in loss of smoothness of its surfaces, and that also can limit joint movements.

Muscles acting on a joint can become weak. This weakness is due to the body's reaction to pain; messages are sent from the brain telling these muscles not to move the painful joint. The muscle weakness and the damage to the joint surfaces also result in joint instability and loss of coordination. Floating cartilage fragments inside the joint can cause pain and further loss of movement. Crackling sounds (crepitus) are often heard when a joint is moved.

**Muscles acting on OA-affected joints become weak
due to the body's reaction to pain, which signals
these muscles to stop contracting.**

The typical person with OA has excessive body weight, is middle-aged or elderly, and complains of pain and stiffness in and around a joint, accompanied by limited physical function. Pain is the key symptom and determines the level of disability or loss of physical function. The pain in the early stages is mild to moderate, gets worse when the joints are used, and is relieved with rest and by taking simple painkillers. As the disease progresses, the pain may increase in intensity and will not be relieved by painkillers or NSAIDs. Pain at rest or during the night is an indication of more severe OA and may be due to joint inflammation. Severe pain can cause interruption of sleep, emotional upset, and poor quality of life.

**Pain at rest or during sleep is an indication
of severe OA and may result in
exhaustion and emotional upset.**

Morning stiffness is common in individuals with OA, but in contrast to the pain and stiffness from rheumatoid arthritis, OA stiffness tends to last less than thirty minutes. People with OA report that they stiffen after sitting or lying for a short period of time, but the stiffness eases once they start to move again.

Most patients assert that the pain and stiffness are affected by changes in the weather, worsening during damp, cool, and rainy days. Affected knee joints tend to buckle and are unstable, especially when a person is descending stairs or stepping off of curbs. OA of the hip joint results in pain in the groin and makes walking, rising from a sitting position, and stair climbing difficult. OA of the hands causes problems with coordination and hand movements (dexterity), especially if the joints near the thumb are involved. Involvement of the joints of the upper spinal column (cervical spine) and lower spinal column (lumbar spine) can press on nerves issuing from the spine on their way to the legs or arms or due to narrowing or stenosis of the spinal canal. This pressure results in neck or low-back pain. Sometimes the pain is felt down the upper and lower extremities (referred pain). The pressure on nerves can also cause weakness in the muscles of the limbs, as well as unusual sensations, such as tingling and loss of skin sensations.

An X-ray of a normal joint will show a space between the joint surfaces, as the cartilage covering the bone ends does not show on X-rays. When the cartilage becomes thinner due to OA, X-rays will show a narrowing or disappearance of this joint space. For this reason, an X-ray of a joint is a very important diagnostic tool for the diagnosis of OA.

Currently, there is no known cure for OA; however, effective treatments are available. The general principles of OA treatment are:

✦ Patient education.

✦ Pain relief.

✦ Maintaining and/or improving function.

✦ Limiting physical disability.

✦ Joint replacement surgery

✦ Weight control.

Patient Education

Basic education about OA is essential so that patients can participate effectively in their care. Self-help books and pamphlets are available from the Arthritis Foundation in the United States, the Arthritis Society in Canada, and sister organizations in other countries. Self-management courses are also helpful, such as the Arthritis Self-Help Program that is available through local chapters of the Arthritis Foundation and The Arthritis Society. Patient education has been shown to improve the results of treatment and reduce the costs of health care. See the resources section of this book for more sources of patient education materials.

Pain Relief

Acetaminophen is recommended in mild cases for the relief of pain. For patients who do not get pain relief from acetaminophen, a course of NSAIDs that also control inflammation, such as ibuprofen, may be used. In patients with severe OA, stronger pain-relieving medication, such as tramadol or, as last resort, painkillers with narcotic ingredients such as codeine, may be prescribed. Non-narcotic pain relief can also be obtained by the application of hot or cold packs. For more information on pain-relief methods and medications, see Chapters 6 and 7.

Maintaining or Improving Function

To maintain or improve function, physical and occupational therapy can be helpful. Exercise to strengthen muscles acting on a joint and other exercise to increase the range of joint movements are essential. Also, general exercises such as aerobics or water aerobics will improve exercise endurance. Assistive devices, such as long-handled shoehorns, walking aids, and shoe insoles, can protect the joints from extra stress and help the patient to conserve energy.

**Joint-replacement surgery can eliminate the
pain of OA and improve the quality of life.**

Joint-replacement surgery has been used effectively to limit pain and improve physical function. These surgeries, especially common for hip and knee joints, can provide symptom relief that may last for twelve to fifteen years. Further information on surgical options is available in Chapter 17.

Weight Control

Individuals with OA who are overweight are encouraged to lose weight in order to reduce stress on joints of the lower limbs. Dietary advice can be obtained from dietitians and self-help books. Before undertaking a weight-control program or going on any serious diet, you should consult your physician.

**If you are overweight and have OA, a loss of
ten pounds can help to reduce knee pain.**

DIFFUSE PAIN SYNDROMES

Diffuse pain syndromes are illnesses characterized by body-wide (diffuse) pain and a range of other symptoms that do not seem to arise from any specific or identifiable cause. These syndromes and other causes of diffuse pain can easily be confused and may overlap to some extent.

Fibromyalgia (FM)

Fibromyalgia, or FM, the most common diffuse pain syndrome, is a chronic condition that does not affect the joints but produces widespread muscular pain and stiffness accompanied by specific tenderness in certain areas of the body, as well as sleep disturbances. Two categories of FM are recognized: primary FM, where there is no significant underlying condition that explains the symptoms; and secondary FM, which occurs in people in conjunction with other diagnosed diseases, such as RA. It is estimated that 1 to 10 percent of the population may have FM; more women than men have the condition. A typical FM patient is a woman, thirty to fifty years of age, who may have seen several health professionals for her complaints, had extensive investigations of symptoms to no avail, and complains of constant generalized pain and fatigue.

A typical patient with FM is a middle-aged woman who complains of generalized pain, fatigue, and lack of sleep.

FM was first noted in nineteenth-century medical literature and was given exotic names such as spinal irritation, Charcot's hysteria, or morbid affection. In the 1970s, physicians began to take note and gave the condition a new label—fibrositis syndrome. It was described as a "psychological phenomenon with physical symptoms that range from pain, fatigue, depression, sleep problems, headaches, irritable bowel, and skin color changes." In 1990, it was again renamed as fibromyalgia syndrome. It is referred to as a syndrome, as it consists of several symptoms that lack clear signs of disease and are not measurable by diagnostic indicators such as blood tests or changes on X-rays.

The cause of FM is unknown; investigations show no consistent abnormalities. Some patients may have experienced a previous injury, infection, or surgery. Other patients may have chronic illnesses such as RA, or they may experience temporary cessation of breathing during sleep (sleep apnea) that causes constant sleep interruption. FM is difficult to diagnose because it is not manifested in blood tests or X-rays, and there are no observable changes in tissues viewed under a microscope. Not all FM patients look the same. The disease is usually diagnosed by a process of elimination as a physician carefully rules out other conditions. Most patients experience poor sleep, fatigue, and generalized pain. Specific areas of the body are tender on pressure and are commonly called "tender points."

The American Rheumatism Association has established guidelines for the diagnosis of FM. Patients who have tenderness in response to pressure exceeding four kilograms, or about nine pounds, at eleven of eighteen designated tender point sites on the right and left sides of the body, are thought to have FM.

There is an ongoing debate among physicians regarding the value of an "official" FM diagnosis. Some do not find the diagnosis of FM helpful, as it condemns patients to viewing themselves as ill, or even feeble, and gives them a reason to label themselves as physically disabled for the rest of their lives. These doctors say that symptoms of FM exist to a varying degree in a lot of people, and labeling those with extreme symptoms as ill and in need of medical care can lead to unnecessary and costly treatments.

**A diagnosis of FM helps rule out other problems
but should not be viewed by sufferers as a "life sentence."**

Other doctors consider a diagnosis of FM as a more useful tool. If someone seems to have FM, it is helpful to rule out other problems. But it is also important to tell the patient that having a diagnosis is no reason to retreat from life's challenges and joys. People with FM can get better, manage their pain, and lead productive lives.

As with other forms of arthritis, successful treatment of FM requires the involvement of a health-care team that may consist of a family physician, a rheumatologist, a physical therapist, a psychologist, and a social worker. Medications usually used to treat arthritis inflammation, such as NSAIDs, or arthritis pain, such as acetaminophen, are not effective for FM pain. Pain medications that include narcotic substances such as codeine are to be avoided, as they can be addictive in the long term. Low doses of antidepressant drugs such as amitriptyline, or muscle relaxants such as cyclobenzaprine, taken early in the evening, may improve sleep, but they are effective in only 30 percent of patients and only for short periods.

Aerobic exercise that increases muscle endurance and fitness is helpful in reducing FM pain and improving the level of functioning. Exercise has also been shown to improve an individual's sense of control over symptoms and general well-being. To benefit from exercise therapy, FM patients must commit to an exercise program and cannot use the excuse that work of any kind makes their pain worse. FM patients should be encouraged to become physically active and also to learn to pace their activities to avoid exhaustion. Walking or exercising in a warm pool (water aerobics) is an excellent choice. Supervised group exercises can help to provide motivation.

Aerobic exercise improves the quality of life among those who suffer from the pain of FM.

FM patients need special coping skills to manage their pain. The Arthritis Self-Management Course, offered by local chapters of the Arthritis Foundation and The Arthritis Society, is commonly used to teach patients coping skills, helping them to reduce their psychological distress and control their pain.

A number of unproven remedies, such as herbal medicines, magnets, and copper bracelets, have been used by FM patients with varying degrees of success. These may offer individuals short-term relief, probably lasting two weeks or less. One way to determine if such a treatment has a true effect on FM symptoms is to begin a course of treatment, then stop if symptoms improve. This will help to determine if the symptoms again get worse once treatment has stopped. Worsening of symptoms after stoppage of treatment could mean that the treatment is effective. Very few unproven remedies meet that test.

While FM is considered by many to be a major health challenge, a diagnosis of FM is no reason to spiral into depression, because much can be done to manage the condition. A positive attitude and disciplined exercise regime can do much to alleviate symptoms.

Looking Forward

This chapter described the most common and severe forms of arthritis and provided a summary of how each can be diagnosed and treated. More detailed treatments for these conditions are provided in the remaining chapters of this book, with special attention given to the physical, social, and psychological effects of these conditions.

Chapter 4

Where Can I Go
For Help?

The first three chapters of this book have explained what arthritis is, the structure and function of human joints, and the various forms of the illness. The following pages present information about what kinds of care and support are available to you if you have arthritis or a related condition. The information is intended to guide you in making choices for managing your arthritis and getting the support you need whether you are experiencing early symptoms or have had arthritis for many years.

What Rights and Responsibilities
Do People with Arthritis Have?

In the United States, the American College of Rheumatology is urging Congress to enact the Arthritis Prevention, Control, and

Cure Act of 2007 in order to "expand efforts to discover and implement new ways to prevent, treat, and care for patients with arthritis and related rheumatic diseases." The act would put into place a national arthritis action plan to increase support for federal and state public-health activities and outreach programs to prevent and manage arthritis. You can read more about it at www.rheumatology.org.

The Arthritis Society in Canada, in consultation with many stakeholders nation-wide, released in 2001 the Bill of Rights for people with arthritis. This bill urges governments and other agencies across Canada to work to develop the Arthritis Strategy. A copy of the Bill of Rights can be found at www.arthritis.ca.

According to the Bill of Rights, people with arthritis have the *right* to:

1. Timely and accurate diagnosis.

2. Timely access to specialty care.

3. Information about arthritis and about their arthritis care.

4. Informed consent regarding treatment decisions.

5. Access to medications and other treatments.

6. Full participation in society (including self-care, leisure, and work pursuits).

7. Research.

8. Representation.

The bill also outlines the responsibilities of people with arthritis. People with arthritis have the *responsibility* to:

1. Pursue healthy lifestyles.

2. Become knowledgeable about their arthritis treatment plans.

3. Actively participate in decisions about their arthritis care.

4. Cooperate fully with mutually accepted courses of treatment.

In North America, thousands of people, patients, professionals, researchers, and government officials have become advocates for prevention, treatment, and education strategies. You may wish to become involved and can learn how by visiting the web sites listed here or by contacting the American College of Rheumatology or The Arthritis Society.

WHEN SHOULD I SEEK HELP?

The onset of arthritis may be sudden and severe, or it may develop slowly over time, affecting just one or two joints at first. Pain, swelling, and stiffness may be constant or periodic. It may strike, for example, only after a particular activity, or after a period of rest. You may feel well apart from the joint discomfort, or you may feel generally unwell and notice a loss of energy.

You should see a health-care provider, usually your family physician, if you experience the following:

✦ Pain in your joints that lasts for more than six weeks.

✦ Stiffness or difficulty moving your joints after a period of rest.

✦ Swelling of any of your joints.

✦ Joint pain that interferes with your ability to carry out your usual activities.

Experts in the treatment of arthritis have come up with the following "red flags" that require urgent medical care:

✦ A history of significant joint injury.

✦ Acute, severe joint pain.

✦ Local or general muscle weakness.

✦ Significant constitutional symptoms, such as fever, weight loss, malaise (flu-like symptoms).

✦ Severe, burning pain or numbness and tingling in the limbs.

✦ A hot and swollen joint.

Pay attention to "red flags!"

Please refer to Figure 3.1, The Flow Chart for Self-Assessment of Arthritis, in Chapter 3, for more assistance with symptom assessment.

HOW CAN I GET THE HELP I NEED?

Because there are more than 120 types of arthritis, knowing which type you may have is the first step toward developing an effective treatment program that suits your individual needs and condition. (See Chapter 3 for more information about the different types of arthritis.) The decisions about your treatment are yours to make. In order to make those decisions wisely, you will want to learn everything you can about your disease and how to manage it.

Take an active role to gain control.

Research studies have shown that people with arthritis who take an active role in the management of their condition have a greater sense of control over their lives, experience less pain, and use the health-care system less frequently. This book is intended to help you to take control over your condition and to become the central figure or leader of your treatment team.

Who Should Be on My Treatment Team?

The problems associated with arthritis may be complex and often affect many aspects of your life. The variety of symptoms that you may experience can mean that several health-care providers may be part of your treatment team at any point in time. You—the patient—are the central focus of a coordinated, multidisciplinary plan of action (Figure 4.1).

You are at the center of your management plan.

In order to protect the public from treatment by unscrupulous or unqualified individuals, states and provinces in North America and elsewhere have regulatory bodies, known as state boards or provincial regulatory colleges. To be licensed by these authorities, health-care providers must meet certain educational requirements and have demonstrated that they have the necessary knowledge, skills, and attitudes to practice within the profession. It is wise, when seeking health care, to make sure that the person offering service is regulated within the state, province, or country in which you live. Remember that you have the right to ask your health-care provider about his or her qualifications and to ask if he or she is a regulated health-care professional. If the health-care provider is regulated, he or she should display a licensing certificate in the clinic or office.

Each health-care professional on the arthritis treatment team featured in Figure 4.1 has a unique combination of knowledge and skills to contribute. Some have skills that overlap with those of other professionals on your team. This means that, at times, you may only need the help of one or two providers, and at other times you may need several. The following is a description of the roles of various providers that constitute the arthritis treatment team. All team members listed below are regulated within their states or provinces.

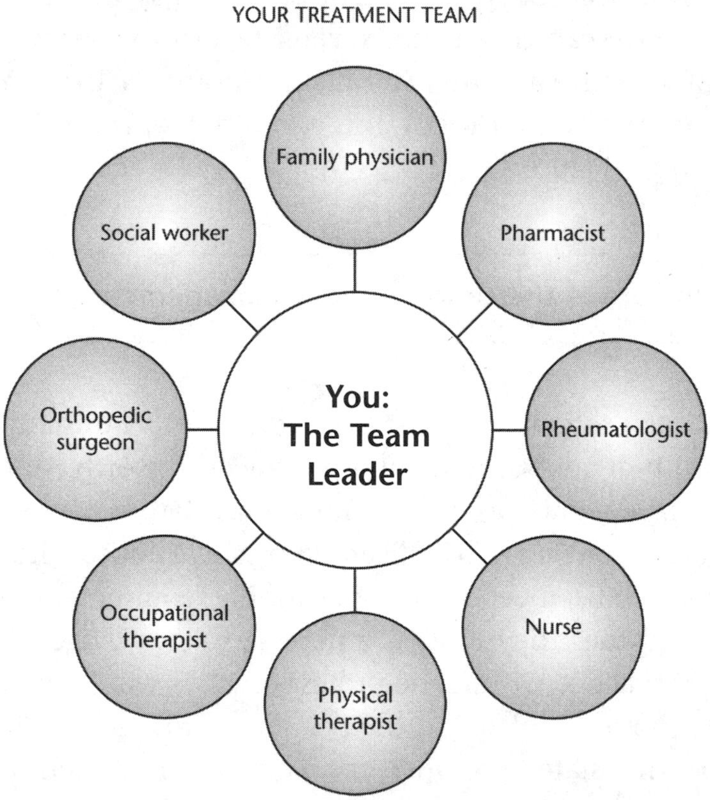

YOUR TREATMENT TEAM

Figure 4.1
You are the leader of your treatment team.

Family Physicians

Usually, people who think they may have arthritis begin by seeing their family physician or primary-care physician. If you are already seeing another type of health-care provider, he or she may suspect that you have arthritis and may suggest that you seek medical care. If you do not have a family physician, this is the time to find one and begin to establish a trusting relationship, because the management of your arthritis may be a long-term process. Family physicians and primary-care physicians work in private practice, community clinics, group practices, and health maintenance organizations. Most are affiliated with at least one hospital.

Your physician should ask you questions about your condition and your general health. If a physician believes that you do have arthritis, he or she will conduct a physical examination and perhaps order certain blood tests and X-rays that can help make a diagnosis. In osteoarthritis, X-rays will exhibit changes to the structure of the joint, such as the loss of the protective cartilage that covers the bone ends. X-rays are taken in order to have baseline information about the state of the joints, especially the hands and feet. If you are experiencing early symptoms of the disease, no significant changes may be apparent, but over time, changes can be more easily monitored once this baseline set of X-rays has been established.

Depending on the type of arthritis you have, your physician may prescribe medications either to ease the pain or to control the inflammation within your joints. It is important for you to know exactly what the medication is expected to do, how soon to expect results, the precise dosage, and what potential side effects may occur. You can read more about arthritis medications in Chapter 6. Your family physician may refer you to a rheumatologist, an orthopedic surgeon, or other professionals, such as a physical therapist, a social worker, or an occupational therapist.

Your health care is your business.

It is your responsibility to be informed about your condition and available treatments. Ask questions! You may want to make a list of questions to take with you to the doctor, because during the visit, many people are nervous, distracted, or upset and forget to ask. The following list can help remind you of the information you need.

✦ What kind of arthritis do I have?

✦ How can I manage the pain of arthritis?

✦ What kinds of medication do I need, and what are the potential side effects, benefits, and risks of these medications?

✦ Do I need to lose weight? Should I eat a special diet?

✦ Where can I get help with my daily activities?

✦ What about exercise?

✦ Do I need to see other health-care providers?

✦ Do I need special equipment, such as canes, splints, or bathroom aids?

Once you have a confirmed diagnosis of arthritis, you will want to learn everything you can about your condition. Keep asking questions, and search out other reliable sources of information other than just your physician. You may want to contact the Arthritis Foundation in the United States or The Arthritis Society in Canada. In addition, these two organizations have sister organizations in other parts of the world. (See the resources section for contact information for these organizations.)

Rheumatologists

For people with the inflammatory types of arthritis, such as rheumatoid arthritis and psoriatic arthritis, and the many related, less common, but potentially serious conditions, a referral to a rheumatologist is usually a first priority. Research has shown that early diagnosis and treatment can prevent long-term joint damage and disability.

Rheumatology is the study of arthritis and other disorders of the joints, ligaments, and muscles. Rheumatologists are physicians trained in internal medicine and specializing in the field of rheumatology. They have special expertise in the diagnosis and treatment of arthritis and other disorders of muscles and ligaments. They are also often involved in teaching and conducting research into the causes and treatments of arthritis.

Sometimes a rheumatologist may see a patient only once, in order to confirm the diagnosis and make recommendations for treatment. He or she will then refer the patient back to the family physician for ongoing treatment. However, patients with progressive inflammatory arthritis, like rheumatoid arthritis, will most likely see a rheumatologist repeatedly. In cases where the arthritis is very active or is complicated by other problems, the patient may be seen frequently to monitor and adjust medications.

In all cases, the rheumatologist should engage in ongoing communication with the other treatment team members, including your doctor. Your rheumatologist, with an in-depth knowledge of rheumatic diseases and a familiarity with the surgeons, occupational and physical therapists, nurses, social workers, and other experts in your community, can help you find the right treatment options at the right time. You, at the center of the team, can then choose the people who can best help you initiate the optimal treatment plan to meet your needs.

Rheumatologists may work in private practice or in arthritis or rheumatic diseases centers associated with university teaching hospitals. A register of rheumatologists in the United States can be found at www.rheumatology.org. In Canada, you can contact university teaching hospitals or the provincial medical association to locate a rheumatologist in your region. Your insurer may require that you be referred by another physician or surgeon before you see a rheumatologist.

Nurses, Nurse Practitioners, and Physician Assistants

Nurses, nurse practitioners, and physician assistants must be registered or licensed in the province or state in which they practice. They must meet certain educational requirements as set out in the legislation of that state or province. Nurses may work alongside rheumatologists, taking medical histories, performing physical examinations, reviewing test results, and administering medications and other treatments. Nurses may be responsible for coordinating the care of the patient and communicating with other team members, as well as providing information to patients, in groups or individually. You can rely on nurses to provide explanations of the ways in which the medications are to be taken, their potential side effects, and what signs and symptoms or other concerns need to be reported to your physician.

In many locations, physician assistants and nurse practitioners with advanced training are available to extend the reach of the physician. Depending on the setting in which they work, physician assistants and nurse practitioners may order various blood tests and X-rays, provide a diagnosis, and make referrals to specialists. The role of the physician assistant or nurse practitioner may differ according to the legislation in various states and provinces.

Nurses, nurse practitioners, and physician assistants work in the rheumatologist's office, in a community clinic setting, in industry, or within a hospital arthritis unit.

Orthopedic Surgeons

Orthopedic surgeons are initially trained as physicians and then go on to be trained in the assessment and surgical management of muscles, bones, and joints. They frequently treat patients with joint damage from osteoarthritis, rheumatoid arthritis, and other types of arthritis.

Surgery may be indicated in situations where your arthritis is causing pain at rest or waking you in the night. If you are unable to work or carry out activities that are necessary in your daily life because of your damaged joints, surgery may help to restore your normal activities. There have been many advances in joint surgery in recent years. Operations such as hip and knee replacements are common and can greatly improve the quality of life of patients. See Chapter 17 for more discussion of surgical options.

If you have been referred to an orthopedic surgeon for surgery, be sure to ask about the risks of the surgery and about what improvements you can expect as a result of the surgery. The following is a suggested list of questions to ask your orthopedic surgeon.

✦ What kind of anesthetic will be used?

✦ Will I need to discontinue any of my current medications?

✦ What will I be able to do after the surgery, and how long is the recovery period?

✦ Will I need help at home following surgery? Is help available within my community? At what cost?

✦ Do I need any equipment, such as a raised toilet seat, canes, or crutches?

✦ Will I need to go to a rehabilitation center or visit a physical therapist?

You might also consider asking if there is a pre-operative education program available, or if you would benefit from seeing a physical therapist or occupational therapist before surgery.

If you are considering surgery, plan ahead for your return home so that your family and friends can be available to assist with transportation to therapy, doctor visits, or help with shopping and errands.

Orthopedic surgeons work in private practice, in group practices, and sometimes on a contract basis for health-maintenance organizations. They also work in hospitals, including hospitals with arthritis units where they are generally a part of the arthritis team. To see an orthopedic surgeon, you may need to be referred by a rheumatologist or your family physician.

Physical Therapists

Physical therapists, known in Canada as physiotherapists, have traditionally been university graduates with a bachelor's degree. More recently, the entry level has been upgraded to a masters-degree level in nearly all jurisdictions in the United States and Canada. Physical therapists study the mechanisms of how the muscles and joints work in daily activities. They also understand how pain affects people and the ways in which various treatments work to relieve pain. They may employ pain-management techniques, such as the application of heat or ice or electrical devices like transcutaneous electrical neuromuscular stimulation (TENS).

When you see a physical therapist (PT), you will be asked questions about your condition and how it is affecting you, what kinds of difficulties you have with normal activities of daily living, and the pain you may be experiencing. A PT will also carry out a full assessment of the state of your joints and muscles to determine whether or not inflammation is present, if the joints are moving through a full range, and if the muscles acting on these joints are working well.

The results of the assessment will help to guide the kind of physical therapy treatment you may receive. You should expect to discuss the goals of the treatment and to decide with the therapist which goals are most important to you. The goals should be Specific, Measurable, Achievable, Realistic, and Time specific (SMART). From there, you and the physical therapist can plan a program for your personal needs.

Set SMART goals!

Physical therapists work with people to develop exercise programs to relieve stiffness, improve movement of the joints, and strengthen the muscles that support the joints. Experts agree that people with arthritis can exercise safely without damaging their joints. Research has also shown that people with arthritis who exercise regularly feel better, emotionally and physically, and report that they have better control over their arthritis. A physical therapist is the best person to help you develop an exercise program that is suited to your individual needs and to advise you about which recreational or sporting activities are likely to be beneficial—and which you should avoid or adapt, depending on how serious your disease may be.

PTs can also educate you about your disease and teach you to use your joints in the most effective and safe way, to save energy by balancing rest and exercise, and how to use devices such as braces or canes to protect your joints and move around more easily.

A physical-therapy program is most successful if you follow the advice of your physical therapist, regularly perform your home exercises, and stay active. Be sure to inform your therapist of any changes in your condition so that he or she can work with you to modify your program if necessary.

Physical therapists can keep you moving.

Physical therapists can help you find other resources within your community, such as gyms and pools, support groups, and equipment and footwear suppliers. They may also refer you to other health-care providers for certain services.

Physical therapists work in private practices, health-maintenance organizations, hospitals, rehabilitation centers, and arthritis centers. A physician referral may be required, depending on regulations in your state or province.

Occupational Therapists

Occupational therapists (OTs) are regulated, university-trained health-care providers with a bachelors degree and, more recently, an entry-level masters degree in all jurisdictions in the United States and Canada. Their role is to improve a patient's ability to carry out the normal activities of daily life. They have in-depth understanding of how your disease can affect all aspects of your life and an ability to analyze various activities in detail. For example, they understand what muscles and joints in the hands are needed to open a jar or turn on a tap. Like physical therapists, they will interview you about the history of your condition, examine affected joints, and ask questions about what kinds of activities you may be finding difficult at home and at work. They will inquire about which activities are most important to you and which are enjoyable or essential.

Energy can be in short supply when you have arthritis, either due to the disease process itself or due to the altered body mechanics that may result in greater expenditure of energy to carry out a task. There are many ways an occupational therapist can help you to adapt to the demands of your disease and help you to balance rest with activity. Often, OTs conduct what is known as a functional assessment—a very detailed questionnaire that asks about various aspects of your life, such as dressing activities, personal care, household management, and your work or leisure activities—in order to understand what activities pose the greatest challenges to you. Together, you can problem-solve and set treatment goals that are mutually agreed upon.

Occupational therapists can also provide prefabricated or custom-fitted splints, such as wrist and hand splints, to support inflamed joints.. They can assess foot problems and either modify footwear with special insoles or with inserts such as arch supports, or they can recommend different types of footwear to better support feet and ankles.

One of the key tasks of an OT is to teach patients about joint protection and energy-conservation techniques. They work with patients to identify ways to make activities easier. They may help you to adapt the way you carry out a given activity, or provide equipment that will protect affected joints from undue strain. For example, they may recommend the purchase of a raised toilet seat to ease the strain on painful, stiff hips or knees, or they may suggest that you pad the handles of kitchen utensils to make them easier to grip.

**OTs can assist you with activities of
daily living at home and at work.**

Occupational therapists can visit the home or workplace and make suggestions about ways to adapt your home or workplace in order to make things easier for you. They can work with you to organize your workspace in the home or workplace so that you can reach things more easily or get up and down from sitting with less difficulty. Often, very simple changes will make a great difference, saving your energy and protecting your joints.

When you see the occupational therapist, go prepared with a list of all the activities that you find difficult to do. Consider which activities are most important to you so that you can discuss them.

Occupational therapists work in private practice, community health-care settings, and rehabilitation settings, including arthritis units within larger hospitals. A physician referral may be required depending on regulations in your state or province.

Social Workers

Social workers usually have a masters of social work (MSW) degree from a university and are generally regulated health professionals, depending on individual state or provincial requirements. Not all states or provinces regulate social workers, although there is widespread support for regulation implementation. You will want to ask about the qualifications of the social worker involved in your care.

Living with arthritis isn't easy. It affects every aspect of your life and can make even simple jobs difficult. It can affect your emotions, relationships, work, and sense of self-worth and independence. It can be frustrating. It is unpredictable; some days you may feel fit, and other days you may feel discouraged and experience a great deal of pain. You may not know where to turn for help.

A social worker can help you and your family to adjust to arthritis and to find resources. You may wish to ask for a referral to a social worker if:

✦ You and your family need support and a better understanding of the ways arthritis is affecting your life.

✦ You feel angry or depressed and need to share your feelings.

✦ You need information about community resources, such as pension-plan benefits, disability benefits, assistance for purchasing drugs, financial assistance, or assistance with housing or transportation.

✦ You need to know about job retraining or assistance in dealing with your employment situation.

Or you may just need to talk to someone about your arthritis problems or find community support or support groups where you can meet people with similar problems and challenges. Social workers are skilled in helping people to find many kinds of support to deal with the challenges posed by day-to-day life with long-term conditions.

**Social workers provide emotional support
and can help you find resources.**

Some community facilities, hospitals, and clinics do not charge for social-work services. The costs of these services may be covered by your employee benefits or by your personal insurance plan. If you wish to explore these services, ask your physician or another health-care provider to refer you.

Social workers are often part of the treatment team in hospitals, arthritis units, clinics, community based-health agencies, and private practices.

Pharmacists

Pharmacists earn a bachelors degree in pharmacy and are registered to practice by the regulatory organizations in their state or province. They have extensive knowledge of medical conditions and medications—how they work, how they interact with other medicines, and what side effects they cause. They work with the treatment team and with patients by providing education about medications, their purpose, and their effects.

When you take a prescription to the drugstore, a pharmacist checks to make sure that the prescription is correct for the diagnosis that you have, ensures that the strength of the medication prescribed is correct, and confirms how long you should take the medication. The pharmacist should also check to make sure that the medication will not cause problems with other conditions or allergies you may have, and he or she should explain how the drug may be affected by food or alcohol or other medications.

Your pharmacist can help you use your medications in the most effective ways so that you get the most benefit from them. You should be provided with information about how the medication is expected to help your particular type of arthritis. When a medication is prescribed for you, it is your responsibility to know the following:

✦ What the medication does.

✦ How often to take the medication and how much to take.

✦ If the medication is not effective immediately, how long it will be before you can expect results.

✦ How long you will be taking this medication.

✦ The side effects that could occur, and what action to take if you do experience side effects.

✦ Whether or not to take the medication with food.

✦ If the medication can be taken with other prescribed or "over-the-counter" medicines.

✦ What to do if you miss a dose.

You can also ask your pharmacist for advice about non-prescription medications, such as herbal remedies, that may be recommended to you by friends or relatives. He or she should be able to advise you about their costs, effectiveness, and possible side effects.

Packaging of medications can sometimes pose a problem, so be sure to ask for a different container if you are having difficulty opening containers. There are also various types of pill containers that allow you to measure out your pills on a daily or weekly basis to make it easier for you to remember when to take your medication.

Carry a list of your current medications with you when you visit your health-care provider and your pharmacist. and be sure to tell them about any problems or side effects you may be experiencing. Chapter 6 has more information about taking arthritis medications.

Pharmacists generally work in retail pharmacies, but many are employed by hospitals, and most arthritis centers have pharmacists to provide consultation and educate patients about medications. Pharmacists dispense medication upon receipt of a prescription from a physician.

Dietitians

When you have arthritis, it is important for you to maintain a healthy lifestyle. Good nutrition is an essential place to begin. People with arthritis may neglect their nutrition because meal preparation can be difficult. People with arthritis may lose weight in the initial onset of the disease, but subsequently they may gain weight because they have become less physically active due to pain and stiffness. An abundance of evidence shows that excess weight causes additional strain on affected joints, particularly hips and knees. It has been shown that even a loss of ten pounds can help to reduce knee pain. Whether you are underweight or overweight, a healthy diet is key to helping you maintain the energy you need to carry on with your life.

A dietitian must have a bachelors degree and be registered with a regulatory body in order to practice. Nutritionists, on the other hand, are educated at a variety of levels and are not generally regulated; therefore, you should ask about their credentials.

A dietitian can be of great assistance if you are concerned about your diet for any reason. Because medications can affect your appetite, you need to be sure that you are getting the proper balance of foods in your diet. Some medications interact with food. Some people on medications may have poor appetites and trouble eating much at any one meal. Some people with arthritis such as scleroderma have trouble swallowing their food, need frequent small meals and need advice regarding foods that are easier to swallow. A dietitian will work with you to plan how calories and vitamins can be spread out through the day so that you get the benefits of a healthy diet no matter what your eating issues are.

People seeking the help of a dietitian are sometimes fearful of being placed on a tasteless, strict program of food that they don't like. The great benefit of working with a dietitian is that he or she can teach you how to make healthy, enjoyable choices that will taste good. Dietitians can also advise you how to simplify shopping and meal preparation. They can help you plan menus that are easy to cook based on your energy and physical limitations and may suggest that you work with an occupational therapist to learn ways to make food preparation easier.

Dietitians work in private practice, in community health-care facilities, and in larger hospitals. A referral to a dietitian may be required depending on the state or province and the facility in which he or she works.

Other Health-Care Providers

There are many other health-care providers who offer services to people with arthritis. Some are regulated; others are not. Table 4.1

provides information on these other providers and the services they contribute.

The professionals listed in Table 4.1 (beginning on the next page) are just a few of the many service providers who may be involved in the treatment of arthritis. There are numerous other unregulated practitioners who may offer services claiming to "cure" arthritis or eliminate pain. Some may help and some may be excessively expensive and ineffective. Some claims made by alternative-care providers may be useless at best and potentially harmful. Whatever your choices in the selection of health-care providers, the first step is to verify that the practitioner is qualified to deliver the care offered and to ask about the scientific evidence that supports the treatment recommended. For more information about alternative health-care providers, see Chapter 18.

There are many health-care resources within the community that can contribute to the success of the treatment program you choose. These are further described in the resources section.

Looking Forward

Chapter 5 will help you to understand and evaluate treatment methods and to make good choices in selecting treatment options. It is designed to help you discern which of the many reports of "treatment breakthroughs," arthritis cures, and new discoveries that are frequently reported in the media may be of benefit to you, and which are nothing more than sensational claims designed to provide false hope and empty your pockets.

Table 4.1
Other Healthcare Providers

PROVIDER	QUALIFICATIONS	SERVICES
Ophthalmologists: Work in private practice, in clinics, and in hospitals.	Physicians who are regulated and specialize in the treatment of eye conditions, which may occur in some forms of arthritis.	Examination and treatment of the eyes, including prescription of medications for eye problems and eye surgical care.
Dermatologists: Work in private practice, in clinics, and in hospitals.	Medical specialists with training in diseases of the skin, such as psoriasis, which is associated with some forms of arthritis.	Assessment and treatment of skin conditions.
Neurologists: Work in private practice, in clinics, and in hospitals.	Medical specialists with training in diagnosis and treatment of diseases of the brain, spinal cord, and nerves.	Assessment, diagnosis, and treatment of disorders of the nervous system.
Orthotists: Work in private practice, in rehabilitation centers, in hospitals, and in retail facilities.	Orthotists are not regulated health professionals. They come from a variety of educational backgrounds and	Assessment of foot problems, fit custom-made insoles and other supports to ensure that the foot is supported

Table 4.1
Other Healthcare Providers (continued)

PROVIDER	QUALIFICATIONS	SERVICES
Orthotists: **(continued)**	are certified in manufacture of mechanical appliances, such as braces, splints, and insoles, to support the function of the limbs.	and the shoe is properly fit. Manufacture custom splints. Doctors, physical therapists, and occupational therapists may refer patients to orthotists for custom-made footwear and supports, as well as for splints.
Chiropodists/ **Podiatrists:** Work in private practice, in clinics, in rehabilitation centers, and in hospitals.	Chiropodists and podiatrists are regulated in most states and provinces. Podiatrists are called doctors of podiatric medicine.	Foot-care services, treatment of infections, corns, calluses, bunions, and toenails. Podiatrists may perform limited forms of foot surgery.
Exercise Therapists/ **Kinesiologists/** **Athletic Therapists:** Work in clinics, in rehabilitation centers, in hospitals, in community health programs, and in fitness facilities.	These therapists are not regulated but frequently work with physical therapists to carry out recommended exercise programs.	Design and oversee exercise classes and fitness programs to increase aerobic fitness or strengthen muscles.

Table 4.1
Other Healthcare Providers (continued)

PROVIDER	QUALIFICATIONS	SERVICES
Massage Therapists: Work in private practice, in rehabilitation facilities, in spas, or in beauty salons.	Regulated in some states and provinces; they are trained in the use of massage. techniques.	Apply massage techniques to the soft tissues of the body to relieve tension and relax muscles.
Chiropractors: Work in private practice, in clinics, in rehabilitation centers, or in fitness facilities.	Regulated in all states and provinces; trained in chiropractic colleges— considered alternative health-care providers.	Assessment and treatment of many disorders. Chiropractors believe that manipulation of the spine, or adjustment, alleviates defective functioning and poor health. A scientific basis supporting this form of treatment for people with arthritis has not been shown.
Naturopaths: Work in private practice, in retail stores, and in "holistic health-care facilities."	Regulated in four Canadian provinces and thirteen states in the United States. Educated in some universities and colleges, depending on the state or province.	Offer a system of healing through the use of "natural" products, such as herbs, supplements, and vitamins, as well as heat, light, and other non-invasive therapies.

Table 4.1
Other Healthcare Providers *(continued)*

PROVIDER	QUALIFICATIONS	SERVICES
Naturopaths: **(continued)**		Believe that their products and services allow the body to heal itself. A scientific basis supporting this form of treatment for people with arthritis has not been shown.
Osteopaths: Work in hospitals, in "holistic health facilities," and in private practice.	Regulated in most U.S. states but in only a few Canadian provinces. They are health practitioners who rely on non-surgical, non-pharmaceutical approaches.	Although there is some variation in the methods utilized by osteopaths, they typically treat the causes of pain and imbalance through manipulation of the soft tissues and joints, similar to chiropractic methods. They see their role as facilitating the body's own powers to heal itself. A scientific basis supporting this form of treatment for people with arthritis has not been shown.

Table 4.1
Other Healthcare Providers (continued)

PROVIDER	QUALIFICATIONS	SERVICES
Acupuncturists: May be trained in traditional Chinese medicine. Work in private practice or in clinics.	Regulated in most U.S. states and in three Canadian provinces. Must be certified by accrediting bodies in the United States and in Canada	Originating in China, acupuncture involves the insertion of fine needles at specific points in the body. This causes energy to flow along invisible lines to correct health or block pain. There is some limited evidence that suggests it may be helpful in osteoarthritis in reducing pain. There appears to be no evidence that acupuncture is effective in the treatment of pain in rheumatoid arthritis.

Chapter 5

How Can Scientific Research Help Me Make Choices?

In the last chapter, we discussed some of the individuals and organizations you can look to for help when you are managing your arthritis. One of the places where many people with arthritis turn to in order to learn more about their disease is their regular news source. When you read the paper, turn on the TV, or scan the radio dial, you may discover new information about arthritis and its treatment. How can this information help you make decisions about your health care?

Staying informed is part of being a competent self-manager. In this chapter, we offer some strategies to help you sort through the issues related to understanding new reports about arthritis. While the amount of information in the media may seem overwhelming at times, a simple screening process can help you know what you need to pay attention to and what you can safely ignore.

HOW CAN I FIGURE OUT WHAT TO LISTEN TO AND WHAT TO IGNORE?

The news media regularly report on so-called "breakthroughs" about one form of arthritis treatment or another, often contradicting previous reports on the same topic. Generally, news organizations obtain these news items at press conferences for scientific meetings or in the form of press releases sent to them by scientific journals and pharmaceutical companies. Less reputable sources may also report miracle cures based on personal testimonials about individual experiences. Miracle cures are often "witnessed" in a dramatic fashion at religious meetings, at religious festivals, or at religious shrines.

It is important to consider the source when you read about new treatments and to think about how the source might stand to gain from the release of the information. When news sources, reputable or not, report on current health topics, many of the parties involved may benefit. Newspapers fill their columns and sell copies. Scientists get free publicity for their work, and that publicity does not go unnoticed by research funding agencies. Religious organizations can increase attendance at services and donations to their mission by claiming to offer miracle cures.

Ironically, patients—the people with the most to gain or lose from the information reported in the media—may not stand to benefit from a lot of the information you see reported in the media, particularly partial, erroneous, or false reports. Many people do not know where to begin to sort through all this media hype. As you encounter stories in the news about arthritis, do you find yourself asking questions like these?

✦ Does this new treatment apply to my arthritis?

✦ Are the results of this new treatment believable?

✦ Can my family physician or specialist help me understand these results?

✦ Is the Internet a reliable source for information about arthritis?

✦ How can I understand the research behind current or new treatments?

The remainder of Chapter 5 provides some background information related to each of these questions.

DOES THIS NEW TREATMENT APPLY TO MY ARTHRITIS?

Recall from Chapter 3 that there are many different forms of arthritis, and any one treatment will not necessarily fit all forms of arthritis. If your family physician or specialist gave you a specific diagnosis, such as rheumatoid arthritis, check if the report you are reading refers to your particular diagnosis. Also keep in mind that most forms of arthritis go through stages. They can be mild at the beginning, eventually progressing to a moderate stage, and finally move on to a more severe stage. Therefore, in addition to making sure that the news report refers to your type of arthritis, check if the treatment reported relates to the specific *stage* of your illness.

Your age and gender are other factors that affect your treatment options. Children with arthritis do not necessarily respond to the same treatments as adults with arthritis, and the elderly respond differently than younger adults. In addition, certain forms of arthritis affect boys differently than girls, and women differently than men. Just because a treatment works for one group does not mean it will always work for another group.

**Children, adults, the elderly, boys or girls,
women or men may respond differently
to the same medication.
What works for one group does not
necessarily work for another.**

Even where you live should factor into how you evaluate reports. Some reports of treatment breakthroughs are based on stories in other countries. A drug approved for treatment in one country may not be approved in another. Individual governments decide which drugs meet their standards for safe use and efficacy. If you think that a reported drug or treatment might be helpful for your particular form of arthritis, check with your family physician or pharmacist to find out if the drug is available or approved in your country, state, or province.

ARE THE RESULTS OF THIS NEW TREATMENT BELIEVABLE?

Media reports about new treatments have a great deal of influence on the public's behavior. Even physicians, nurses, pharmacists, physical therapists, and other health professionals look to the news media for the latest developments or controversies that could be of concern to their patients. A new treatment usually receives much publicity, particularly if it concerns a disease for which there is currently no cure, such as rheumatoid arthritis. The accuracy of these reports depends very much on the reporting standards of the source. Given the power they exercise, the media have a responsibility to produce fair, balanced, and well-informed health stories.

**Sometimes it seems like there is a preference
to report unusual or bizarre stories in the
media, especially in the tabloids.**

However, not all media sources take that responsibility equally seriously. Stories of a new breakthrough often are not reported in the same way by all sources. Sometimes it can seem that there is preference in the media to report unusual or bizarre stories—stories that discredit well-known people, or stories about extreme remedies. In certain kinds of media, like supermarket tabloids or sensational talk radio programs, that can often be the case. Even in more reputable papers, reporters complain that space and time constraints imposed by editors, and the flood of competing stories, may reduce a report on a new treatment to the bare essentials.

Given this, it is hard to know what information to trust or believe. However, there are some strategies you can use to screen media information. Here are some ways to make sure that the report you are reading is reliable:

✦ There is safety in numbers. If a number of major mainstream media sources are reporting the same story, it is more likely to be accurate and reliable. For example, reports on new drugs seen in the *New York Times* or on CNN are more likely to be complete and balanced than reports of the same drug seen in pulp tabloids. Important findings are almost always reported in more than one source. Most legitimate developments in arthritis treatment will receive plenty of media attention and be widely reported. If you have access to a computer, you can use a good Internet search engine to make sure if a new treatment is being widely reported in the mainstream media.

◆ When you are reading about new drugs, check to see if the drug is in a phase I, phase II, or phase III trial. All drugs have to meet the requirements of all three phases before they are released for public use. Only phase III drugs have made it through enough of the experimental process to be truly promising; results from phase I and phase II trials, however initially promising, may never pan out. Until a drug reaches phase III trials, it is not worth investing too much attention in it.

◆ Be on the lookout for conflicts of interest between those who research the treatment and the companies that might stand to benefit. For example, drug research is done by independent, well-known research teams at universities or teaching hospitals, but it is usually financed by pharmaceutical companies. Inevitably, researchers keen on getting research funds may be influenced directly or indirectly to report good results. Sometimes new drugs that are not effective can slip through the net of government monitoring agencies and be reported as beneficial. If a result seems too good to be true, and the agency that is reporting the results stands to gain from a positive report, view any findings critically.

◆ Check to see if there is any mention of side effects to this new treatment. Early or suspect reports mention beneficial effects and rarely side effects. However, any legitimate drug producer must inform users of potential side effects. If side effects are not mentioned in detailed articles, then most likely the drug or treatment has not been tested thoroughly by a government agency. Thus, any reports on its efficacy may not be believable. Drug companies are required to monitor side effects, as reported to them by prescribing physicians. Except for drugs to treat life-threatening diseases or extreme pain, it may be prudent to wait a year or two before taking a new drug to see if any new side effects develop in users.

Above all, if you believe for any reason that the report you are hearing is not accurate or reliable, do some double checking to see if you can find out more about the story. Concern about the accuracy of newspaper reports of treatment breakthroughs has led to the creation of Media Doctor in Australia, a web site that provides a fair assessment of articles in the lay press regarding new treatments, drugs, procedures, or diagnostic tests. Canada also now has its own Media Doctor, which can be accessed online at www.mediadoctor.ca. And, most important of course, before you pursue any new treatment option, check with key members of your health-care team, like your physician.

CAN MY FAMILY PHYSICIAN OR SPECIALIST HELP ME UNDERSTAND THESE RESULTS?

Not all family physicians read the journals that report new drugs; those that do have to search for information that may be buried in thousands and thousands of journals. You should not be surprised if your primary-care physician and pharmacist are not familiar with a new drug or other treatment that you mention to them. They also may not be able to immediately tell you if the treatment is a viable option for you. In fact, unless they have obtained advance knowledge from medical journals or reports of scientific meetings, initially your physician and pharmacist may only be able to superficially interpret what is in any report. Health-care professionals have drug directories at their disposal that provide information on all drugs, and although these directories are updated annually, they are unlikely to report a new drug that has just become available on the market.

**If your physician can't answer all your
questions about a new treatment, he or she
should be able to direct you to someone who can.**

Another factor to be aware of is that drug companies spend lots of money on advertising aimed at physicians, hoping to influence what medications are prescribed. Most of us assume—or at least hope—that our physicians are smart enough to see through the sales hype and pick the drug that meets our needs. But what if the pharmaceutical firms are providing physicians with misleading or inaccurate information? This is when the drug company sales representative comes into the picture, supplying charts, extensive "fact" sheets, and samples of the new drug. The information that he or she provides is based on the beneficial effects of the drug at this early stage but is also geared toward helping the company sell more products. Your physician faces a dilemma: He or she must find time to read these reports or journal articles and interpret their scientific results, or he or she can rely on the briefing provided by the drug company representative. Unfortunately, due to the many demands on the time of health-care providers, the briefing of the sales rep may win the day in some cases. As a result, your primary-care physician may sometimes be responding to somewhat biased information when he or she chooses drugs for patients.

**Medical specialists regularly read the journals
that report research results in their specialty.**

The good news is that specialists are generally more discriminating and regularly read the journals that report research results in their specialty. For example, rheumatologists regularly read *The Journal of Rheumatology*, as well as a dozen other relevant journals. Their specialization allows them to focus on new findings about drugs and treatments related to their specialty. Family physicians, as generalists, have a tougher time keeping up-to-date, and a good family physician faced with a problem that is beyond his or her scope should refer you to the appropriate specialist. A pharmacist can also be helpful, as he or she sometimes knows more than a family physician about the ingredients of a given drug, its effects, and its side effects.

The bottom line is, if a reported finding about arthritis is legitimate, someone on your health-care team should be able to tell you more about it. When you read articles about new drugs or treatments, cut them out or copy down the details. If your physician can't answer your questions about the treatment, then he or she should be able to refer you to someone who can—be it another physician, a specialist, or even a knowledgeable pharmacist. If information about a treatment or a drug is not legitimate, your physician or someone else on your health-care team should be able to tell you that as well.

IS THE INTERNET A RELIABLE SOURCE FOR INFORMATION ABOUT ARTHRITIS?

Most consumers know how to evaluate the material in mainstream media, but to many people, the Internet is a whole new world. If you have access to the Internet, you can find a great deal of information about new treatments or new drugs online. Internet

reports tend to be based on the same sources of information reported in the traditional media and therefore have similar limitations.

**When you are surfing the Web for information,
use the same critical thinking skills you employ
when you read the newspaper or watch TV.**

When you read something on the Internet, interpret it the
same way you would a report in the traditional media. Carefully
consider the source of the information. Some of the information
on the Internet follows no particular rules or standards of reporting and therefore can be less reliable than reports in the media and
grossly misleading. However, many reputable news sources and
health-care organizations also have web sites, so there is also excellent, reliable information available online. Still, the average consumer may have a hard time discriminating between fact and
fiction when staring at a computer screen. The following rules may
help.

✦ Get your information from the official web sites of well-regard-
   ed voluntary or public organizations such as the Arthritis
   Foundation in the United States (www.arthritis.org) or The
   Arthritis Society in Canada (www.arthritis.ca). On these web
   sites, you will find information on specific arthritis diagnostic
   groups, such as rheumatoid arthritis, psoriatic arthritis, juvenile arthritis, ankylosing spondylitis, osteoarthritis, and so on.
   These web sites provide comprehensive, balanced information
   and are funded by voluntary organizations that operate at
   arm's length from drug companies and manufacturers of assistive devices. You will also find useful and reliable information

in the consumer's section of the Cochrane Collaboration (www.cochrane.org) by clicking on "arthritis." The collaboration is an international not-for-profit organization providing up-to-date and reliable information on the effects of treatments. In the United States, web site addresses ending in ".gov" are used for official governmental, non-commercial sites. Check the resources section of this book for recommended web sites.

✦ Be wary of information contained in the web sites of drug companies and device manufacturers. Remember that their primary objective is to sell their products, not necessarily to educate the consumer. Drug companies use the Internet and the media extensively in order to sell their over-the-counter or prescription drugs to consumers. Some drug companies have created "patient-advocacy groups" web sites, have launched patient-education campaigns, and have enlisted paid celebrities who are willing to share their stories online. If a spokesperson is being paid, you should not completely believe what that person is saying about a product or cure.

✦ Be sure that what you are reading is scientific reporting, not personal opinion. Information in chat rooms or on blogs can be interesting, but it generally deals with personal experiences that may or may not apply to your condition or disease stage. While the Internet can be a great way to keep in touch with others who share your diagnosis, it can also be a forum for uneducated people to spout unfounded opinions.

The Internet is a valuable source of information sharing, but to find good information online, you have to be selective in your search.

HOW CAN I UNDERSTAND THE RESEARCH BEHIND CURRENT OR NEW TREATMENTS?

Media reports rarely mention or describe the research methods used to study new treatments. But it is important for you to know the procedures used to conduct research or put a study together, as this will have a great deal of bearing on its importance or credibility. Treatment studies use a number of different designs based on field conditions and availability of resources. The remainder of this chapter introduces some of the common approaches used in the study of diseases or new treatments. Knowing what the types of research you read and hear about are and how different studies are conducted will help you to know how much credibility to give the results they produce. Reliable results come only from reliable studies. Please keep in mind as you read this material that for simplicity we will use the terms study, trial, and experiment interchangeably.

Surveys, Cross-Sectional Studies, and Longitudinal Studies

If a researcher has limited time or money to carry on a complex project, only a small number of available patients to enroll in the study, or no experts in the setting to help design a rigorous study, he or she may conduct a *survey*. A survey is also called a *cross-sectional study,* and its purpose is to obtain limited information about the frequency and characteristics of a disease in a population at a particular point in time. This type of study is similar to a public-opinion poll and in the past has been useful in discovering new diseases among groups of similar patients.

The alternative to a survey or cross-sectional study is a *longitudinal study*. A longitudinal study involves observations of the same factors over longer periods of time, often many decades. Longitudinal studies may be used in medicine to figure out predictors of certain diseases.

N of 1 Studies and Before-After Studies

Whenever a patient sees a health-care professional, he or she is evaluated in order to establish what is ailing him or her. Once that is determined, he or she will be prescribed a treatment, and a few days or weeks later, the patient will be evaluated again to find out if the treatment is working. This is like a mini study of one patient, often called an *N of 1 study*. In order to find out if the treatment in an N of 1 study really works, and that any improvements are not just coincidental or due to other factors, a physician may subsequently stop the treatment for a short period of time and monitor the patient's progress. If the patient gets worse when treatment ceases and then gets better again after resuming treatment, it indicates that the treatment is having a positive effect on the patient.

Similarly, a researcher may decide to test a certain treatment with a defined group of patients, then measure its effect on these same patients over the course of three or four months. This is called a *before-after study*. If the patients improve, it means that the treatment has some promise. But, of course, patients may improve over time with or without treatment. Therefore, in this kind of study, it is difficult to tell if other factors are involved or if the treatment is effective.

Case-Control Studies

A *case-control study* is used to find if a certain illness is common in a group of patients who have all been exposed to a potential hazard. Here, the patients exposed to the hazard are compared to another group of individuals of the same age and sex who have not been exposed. This type of study was used to verify the serious effects of exposure to asbestos dust.

> **The findings of a study are only as reliable
> as the methods used to arrive at the findings.**

Cohort Analytical Studies

A researcher may want to compare, over a specified period of time, a new treatment with an old treatment, or compare a new treatment to no treatment or to a placebo. A placebo is an inactive substance or preparation used as a control in an experiment. People who are given the placebo are led to believe it is the real drug; in this way, experimenters can determine whether a result is due to the patient's expectations about the treatment or the actual effects of the treatment.

In a *cohort analytical study*, patients choose which treatment group they will join. Because patients are self-selecting and are not assigned at random to each group in these studies, patients in each group may differ significantly in their age, their sex, their education, and/or their income levels, making like-to-like comparisons difficult between those who receive the treatment and those who do not. In other words, in a study like this, it is difficult to sort out if differences in results arise because of the efficacy of treatments or because the people in the studies were different to begin with.

Double-Blind, Randomized Controlled Trials

The gold standard of research design is the experimental approach referred to as *double-blind, randomized controlled trials.* In this type of study, different treatments are compared; for example, a new treatment versus an older one or a new treatment versus a placebo. What is distinctive about this design is that patients are assigned to treatment groups at random, and researchers can be sure that differences in the results are due to the different treatments each group receives.

Another key feature of this type of trial is that patients do not know to which group they are assigned. The workers who choose and evaluate subject progress also do not know to which group each patient belongs. This is what the term "double blind" means. Because neither the subject nor the researchers know what group patients belong to, they are less likely to report what they expect to happen and to report what really happens.

The most credible research findings come from double-blind, randomized controlled trials.

This type of study is referred to as controlled because there is a *control* group that is established at the outset of the test. A control group is a group of subjects that are as similar to the experimental group as possible except for the fact that they are not being treated. When effects are reported in the treatment group, they can be compared to results for the control group. Researchers are then able to determine if the results are due to the treatment or to other factors.

In this type of study, all factors that can affect results are carefully monitored: how patients are selected and assigned to groups; how they are assessed on admission to the study and at its conclusion; what treatments, dosage, and dosage administration they receive; and what statistical methods are used to analyze the results. A story about a new treatment that refers to this kind of study indicates that the research design and methods used are the finest and most reliable.

Meta-Analysis

Investigators searching for studies related to a particular treatment may find that dozens of studies have previously been published on that topic. Some studies may indicate that the treatment works, while others may not. In order to sort out what is happening in this type of circumstance, a new method of evaluating published studies was developed. It involves lumping all like studies together and analyzing the data as if they were collected from a single study. This "lumping together" increases the number of research subjects in the total pool. This is an advantage, because the more people who are in a study, the more significant its results tend to be. This type of study is called a *meta-analysis*; it is commonly used to mine the results of studies that otherwise would have been inconclusive.

Looking Forward

Patients with arthritis can benefit from being educated consumers and staying well informed about the research that is being conducted on their illness and its treatment. In particular, arthritis patients should pay attention to stories about the effects of new drugs or treatments. For example, you may have read in recent years about the drugs Vioxx and Bextra. These drugs were taken out of circulation after four years of use due to their serious side effects on heart function. The side effects were reported in the *New England Journal of Medicine* three years before the drugs were taken off the market, but no one paid much attention until much later, when heart problems became more widespread in users. When more evidence surfaced, those drugs were removed from pharmacy shelves worldwide, and currently a number of civil suits against the drug companies are pending.

The intention of this chapter is not to discourage arthritis patients from using new treatments or prescription drugs, but to help them take the necessary precautions before they swallow a new pill or accept a new treatment just because the media say it's a "breakthrough" or "cure." In the next chapter, we will discuss more about the medications that are being used to treat arthritis, their mode of operation, their benefits, and their side effects.

Chapter 6

How Can Arthritis Medications Help Me?

In the last chapter, we discussed how arthritis research can direct-ly affect you and your diagnosis. If you pay any attention to the media at all, you will have noticed that much of the research relat-ing to arthritis is focused on new drug treatments. Drug therapy (to treat joint inflammation), in conjunction with physical and occupational therapy (to increase mobility), is at the core of arthri-tis management. Billions of dollars are spent by pharmaceutical companies on research and development of new arthritis-related medications, making very clear the emphasis the medical estab-lishment places on the role of drugs in the management of this group of diseases.

WHAT IS MY ROLE IN
THE PRESCRIPTION PROCESS?

Arthritis is caused by a number of factors, making drug treatment a complicated affair and often requiring that the patient take several drugs simultaneously. While drug treatment can sometimes be beneficial, at other times it can be harmful. The patient and prescribing physician must carefully monitor beneficial or harmful effects of any medication. A recent survey showed that physicians prescribing new medications to a patient typically spend two minutes or less informing the patient about side effects and possible risks with the medication. A quarter of the patients in this study received no counseling at all!

The results of this research underline the importance of your role in the medication conversation. You must ask questions about any new drug that your physician prescribes for you. It is incumbent upon you to ask about its possible side effects as well as the risks of not taking the drug. Be sure that you understand the instructions given by your physician or pharmacist. And always carefully read the printed pamphlet provided by the pharmacist.

In addition to information provided by your physician and pharmacist, this chapter will serve as a resource you can trust—one you can go to in order to make sure that when your physician hands you a prescription for your arthritis, you are well prepared to ask relevant and important questions regarding the medication.

In the following sections, we discuss the relationship of the drug companies to research efforts, outline the role of medication in treating arthritis, tell you what you should know before taking a medication, and discuss prescribing habits of physicians. To help you make sense of the choices you must make about medications, we outline in table form the drug categories and their names, the effects and side effects of a number of common drugs currently available to treat the various forms of arthritis, and the necessary precautions you should observe with these drugs. We also discuss novel drugs that are currently undergoing evaluation and that may provide better control of inflammation with fewer side effects.

WHAT IS THE RELATIONSHIP BETWEEN RESEARCH AND COMMERCE?

The costly investments in new drug research made by drug companies are passed on to the consumer directly in the form of high costs of new drug treatments. But without these expensive clinical trials, there would be no new "miracle" treatments. Without funding from the drug companies, researchers could not test the benefits, safety, or anything else about potential new drug treatments. As a result, new drugs would never reach the market. If the drug company is lucky, its investments yield an expensive, marketable product that patients with chronic diseases must use continuously. Thus, in the best-case scenario, the pharmaceutical company profits and the patient receives better treatment.

In contrast to the big-business budgets of new medicine investment, a fraction of the amount spent on testing new drugs is spent on research and development of so-called orphan therapies, such as physical and occupational therapy. The disparity is due to the fact that physical and occupational therapy treatments (products) are generally not marketable, profit-generating products requiring continuous consumer investment. Thus, it is no surprise that we hear more about the drugs than about the other therapies. But it is equally important that rehabilitation treatments are tested for their safety and effectiveness—first, to avoid harm to the patient, and second, to determine their effectiveness.

WHAT RESPONSIBILITIES DO I HAVE WHEN I TAKE A MEDICATION?

Some medicines may interact with each other. Therefore, you should inform your physician or pharmacist of all prescriptions or over-the-counter medicines that you are taking, including any supplements or herbal remedies. Do not start or stop any medicine without the approval of your physician or pharmacist. Read and follow the instructions given in pamphlet form by your pharmacist regarding medications.

Follow all the instructions for taking a particular medicine provided by your physician. Some medicines may be taken on an empty stomach; others should be taken with food. Unless otherwise instructed by your physician, continue to take the medicine even if you feel well. Do not miss any doses. Do not share your medicine with others. Do not use a medication to treat a health condition for which it was not prescribed. Certain medicines must be taken more carefully by elderly people, because they may be more sensitive to the effects of the medicine.

If your symptoms do not improve, or if they worsen, inform your physician immediately. If you will be taking a medicine for an extended period of time, obtain necessary refills before your supply runs out. If you accidentally take an overdose of the medicine, contact your local poison-control center or hospital emergency department.

Read about any possible side effects that may occur while taking a particular medication in the pamphlet provided by your pharmacist. Check with your doctor if you experience any of these side effects. For certain powerful medications used to treat arthritis, such as methotrexate, the side effects can be very serious and must be dealt with at the earliest opportunity.

For women who plan on becoming pregnant, discuss with your physician or pharmacist the benefits or risks of taking this medicine during pregnancy, as certain medicines can affect the fetus. Some drugs are excreted in breast milk, so you need to be aware of this if you plan to breast-feed while taking medicines.

Most medicines need to be stored at room temperature in tightly closed containers, away from heat or light. The container should be childproof but easy to open for arthritis patients. You may be required to cut certain pills in half in order to obtain the correct dose. If a tablet is scored or has a groove running down the middle, it is made that way so that it can be safely split, but this can cause a problem for the elderly or people with hand arthritis. Ask your pharmacist to do the splitting if the pills are spindle-shaped; if they are round or octagonal, invest in a tablet cutter, which should be available at your local pharmacy at very little cost. If a tablet is not scored, splitting it is not advisable as the drugs concentration is not uniform in the tablet.

Most tablets that can be cut are also safe to crush, but check with your pharmacist before doing so. To crush a tablet, place it in a small, clear plastic bag, and crush the tablet with the back of a spoon. If the medication is in capsule form and opens easily, it is usually acceptable to open it and mix the contents with water, as long as you drink the mixture immediately. In general, any tablet that has a gel coating should not be split or crushed. If a capsule is sealed, it should probably stay that way. Sealed capsules or pills that are formulated to release a drug into your bloodstream slowly throughout the day (time-release medications) should never be split or crushed. If you are not sure whether a medication is time-released, speak to your physician or pharmacist before opening, breaking, or crushing it.

Taking your medicines at the same time each day can help you remember to take them. For arthritis patients, missing a dose here and there is not a life-threatening situation, but it can reduce the effectiveness of the medication, leaving you vulnerable to joint inflammation. The main exception to this rule is prednisone. If you do not take your scheduled doses of this drug, you may experience weakness, loss of appetite, nausea, low blood pressure, and/or dizziness. If you miss a dose of any medication, you should take it as soon as possible, unless it is very close to the time you were to take the next dose. In that case, wait until your normal next-dose time, skipping the missed dose entirely, and get back on schedule. To regulate your dosing schedule, invest in an inexpensive, daily-medication organizer. These are available at your local pharmacy and will help you remember to take the right dose of your medications at the right time.

The length of time between when you take your first dose of medicine and when you experience its effects can vary widely—from a matter of minutes to a matter of months. How long it takes for a drug to work depends on your body makeup, the benefits you are seeking, and the drug itself. For example, it takes longer to reduce joint inflammation than it does to lower a fever or ease mild pain.

A Word About Off-Label Prescribing

Pharmaceutical firms go to great expense to get drugs approved for treating specific conditions. Once a drug is on the market, however, physicians are free to prescribe it for any condition they want. The practice, known as "off-label prescribing," gives physicians a lot of flexibility in treating certain conditions. Numerous drugs are used for a variety of conditions beyond those for which they were first developed and tested. A recent study showed that 21 percent of medications were prescribed for off-label uses, and of these off-label prescriptions, 73 percent lacked scientific support. In other words, in those cases, there had been no documented research done on the effectiveness of prescribing that particular drug for the "off-label" condition. Many consumer advocates agree that government regulators and pharmaceutical companies need to do a better job of monitoring off-label prescribing. Upon receiving a new prescription, check with your physician or pharmacist if the medicine prescribed has been first approved by government regulators for your particular condition, and if not, whether there is solid scientific support for its off-label use.

A Word About Drug Names

Keep in mind that each drug has a brand name given to it by the company that manufactured that drug, and a generic name that is not protected by a trademark. For example, take Motrin, a well-known anti-inflammatory drug for arthritis. Motrin is this drug's brand name; its generic name is ibuprofen. Media reports of new drugs often refer to brand names, because new drugs are initially developed and marketed by the pharmaceutical companies who name them. However, after the initial development and advertising period, generic names are more typically used. When the patent on a brand-name drug lapses, several other manufacturers can produce it and sell it under its generic name only. Your physician may prescribe a drug under either its brand name, which usually costs considerably more, or in its less-costly generic version. Generic drugs must meet the same government standards as brand-name drugs, and some health-insurance companies will pay only for generic drugs because they are less expensive.

WHAT ROLE DO MEDICATIONS PLAY IN ARTHRITIS TREATMENT?

Medication may be prescribed to arthritis patients for one or more of the following reasons:

✦ To decrease joint pain.

✦ To control joint inflammation.

✦ To prevent disease progression.

How these objectives are fulfilled depends on the type of arthritis present and how it is affecting the patient. Several forms of arthritis may be treated with the same drugs if they share similar symptoms. Other forms of arthritis are treated with one or more drugs that are unique to these conditions alone. During the last few years, for certain forms of arthritis (such as rheumatoid arthritis), in which the immune system is affected, powerful drugs such as methotrexate have been prescribed to patients the moment they are diagnosed. These drugs are meant to be taken together with less powerful anti-inflammatory drugs such as Naproxen, as well as pain-relieving drugs such as Tylenol. In contrast, for osteoarthritis, in which pain is the dominant symptom, pain-relieving drugs are typically the only drugs prescribed upon the initial diagnosis.

A GUIDE TO ARTHRITIS MEDICATIONS

This section is to be used as a reference to medications that you would like to know more about. These may include the medications you already are taking as well as new medications you might like to consult about with your physician to see if they would be worth trying. Knowing more about arthritis medications will help you take an active role in your arthritis treatment and make sense of your medication cabinet.

The medications in Tables 6.1 to 6.6 are identified by their generic name, which is shown in the first column. Where applicable, the brand name (the name given by the manufacturer) in the United States or Canada is listed in parentheses below the generic name.

In the tables, the medications are grouped according to the effect they will have on your arthritis. Pain-relieving drugs, also known as analgesics and nonsteroidal anti-inflammatory drugs (NSAIDs), form one group (Table 6.1). Disease-modifying, anti-rheumatic drugs (DMARDs) make up the second group (Table 6.2). Biologic response modifiers (BRMs), which function similarly to DMARDs, are a third group (Table 6.3). Corticosteroids form the fourth group (Table 6.4). These are the four groups of drugs commonly used to treat inflammatory and degenerative joint disease. Specific medications used in the treatment of fibromyalgia and gout are included as groups five (Table 6.5) and six (Table 6.6), respectively.

Analgesics

Pain is a potentially debilitating symptom of arthritis, and for many patients, pain relief is the most important priority. Fortunately, many of the drugs, such as analgesics (in Table 6.1), which are used to treat inflammation and slow disease progression, relieve pain as well.

Table 6.1
Analgesics and Nonsteroidal Anti-inflammatory Drugs (NSAIDs)

**ANALGESICS AND NONSTEROIDAL
ANTI-INFLAMMATORY DRUGS, OR NSAIDS**

Uses/Effects	Side Effects	Monitoring
Analgesics relieve pain; NSAIDs relieve pain and reduce inflammation.	Upset stomach, peptic ulcer, bleeding, renal (kidney) failure. Use of NSAIDs may increase the rate of miscarriage in pregnant women.	Before taking these drugs, let your physician know if you drink alcohol or use blood thinners or if you have any of the following: sensitivity or allergy to aspirin or similar drugs, kidney or liver disease, heart disease, high blood pressure, asthma, or peptic ulcer.

**ACETAMINOPHEN (ANACIN, EXCEDRIN,
PANADOL, TYLENOL, TYLENOL ARTHRITIS)**

Uses/Effects	Side Effects	Monitoring
Non-prescription medication used to relieve pain.	Usually no side effects when taken as directed.	Not to be taken with alcohol or with other products containing acetaminophen.

Table 6.1
Analgesics and Nonsteroidal Anti-inflammatory Drugs (NSAIDs)
(continued)

ACETAMINOPHEN (ANACIN, EXCEDRIN, PANADOL, TYLENOL, TYLENOL ARTHRITIS) (continued)

Uses/Effects	Side Effects	Monitoring
		Not to be used for more than 10 days in a row unless directed by a physician.

ASPIRIN

Uses/Effects	Side Effects	Monitoring
Aspirin is non-prescription. Buffered or plain, it is used to reduce pain, swelling, and inflammation, allowing patients to move more easily and carry out normal activities. It is generally part of early and ongoing treatment.	Upset stomach, tendency to bruise easily, ulcers, diarrhea, headache heartburn or indigestion, nausea or vomiting.	Physician monitoring is needed.

Table 6.1
Analgesics and Nonsteroidal Anti-inflammatory Drugs (NSAIDs)
(continued)

TRADITIONAL NSAIDS (IBUPROFEN, KETOPROFEN, NAPROXEN, ETC.)

Uses/Effects	Side Effects	Monitoring
NSAIDs such as ibuprofen, ketoprofen, and naproxen help relieve pain within hours of administration, but it may be several days before they reduce inflammation.	For NSAIDs: Abdominal or stomach cramps, pain or discomfort; diarrhea; dizziness; drowsiness or lightheadedness; heartburn or indigestion; peptic ulcers; nausea or vomiting; rarely kidney or liver damage.	For all NSAIDs: Before taking these drugs, let your physician know if you drink alcohol or use blood thinners or if you have or have had any of the following: sensitivity or allergy to aspirin or similar drugs, kidney or liver disease, heart disease, high blood pressure, asthma, or peptic ulcer.

COX-2 INHIBITORS (CELECOXIB, CELEBREX)

Uses/Effects	Side Effects	Monitoring
COX-2 inhibitors, like the other more traditionally administered NSAIDS, block COX-2, an	Stomach irritation, ulceration, and bleeding may occur. Caution is advisable for patients with a	Use of COX-2s with low-dose aspirin is permitted but may slightly increase risk of ulcer.

Table 6.1
Analgesics and Nonsteroidal Anti-inflammatory Drugs (NSAIDs)
(continued)

COX-2 INHIBITORS (CELECOXIB, CELEBREX) (continued)

Uses/Effects	Side Effects	Monitoring
enzyme in the body that stimulates an inflammatory response. Unlike the other NSAIDs, however, they do not block the action of COX-1, an enzyme that protects the stomach lining. This results in reduced risk of gastrointestinal ulceration and bleeding. Reduces joint pain and inflammation.	history of bleeding or ulcers, decreased renal function, hepatic disease, hypertension, or asthma.	Physician monitoring is recommended before taking a COX-2 inhibitor, especially if you have had a heart attack, stroke, angina, blood clot, hypertension, or sensitivity to aspirin or other NSAIDs. Physician monitoring for possible allergic responses to COX-2s is important.

Acetaminophen

Acetaminophen, the most commonly used analgesic, is available under a variety of brand names (Anacin, Panadol, Excedrin, and Tylenol) and does not require a prescription. It is recommended as a first-line drug for treating osteoarthritis pain. Acetaminophen may also be combined with other more powerful pain-relieving drugs such codeine, hydrocodone, or tramadol, as well as other analgesics once reserved for severe pain following surgery, cancer, or traumatic injuries (see Table 6.1). Acetaminophen does not control inflammation, yet recent studies suggest that it controls arthritis pain as effectively as NSAIDs. In some situations, analgesics, when combined with NSAIDs, may relieve pain better than each alone.

Topical Analgesics

Topical analgesics (medications that you rub directly on painful areas) also relieve pain. They are sometimes used when the pain is mild, when a few joints are involved, or when oral medications do not completely relieve your pain. However, they are not a substitute for oral analgesics or NSAIDs. Topical analgesics are not listed in the tables in Chapter 6; instead, they are covered here in the text.

Topical analgesics are available in cream, gel, or salve form and work in one or more of the following ways:

✦ By blocking the transmission of the naturally occurring, pain-relaying substance, called substance P, to the brain. The main ingredient that does this comes from cayenne peppers and is available under several brand names, including Zostrix, Zostrix HP, and Capzasin P.

✦ By creating a feeling of intense cold or heat over sore muscles, thus masking the pain sensations. Appropriately named, counterirritants, such as menthol oil, oil of wintergreen, camphor, eucalyptus oil, and turpentine oil, work this way. Counter-irritant brands include Arthricare, Eucalyptamint, Icy Hot, and Therapeutic Mineral Ice. Menthacin includes both cayenne peppers and counterirritants.

✦ By seeping through the skin to inhibit pain and inflammation. The main ingredients in substances that work this way are sal-icylates, available in over-the-counter products like Aspercreme, BenGay, Flexall, Mobisil, and Sportscreme.

Non-Steroidal, Anti-Inflammatory Drugs (NSAIDs)

NSAIDs are the most widely used drugs in arthritis. They control joint inflammation and, in doing so, also relieve pain. At low doses, they also help relieve headaches, muscle aches, minor pain, and fever. There are about twenty generic NSAIDs; the most com-monly used are listed together with analgesics in Table 6.1. All of these, except for three, are available without a physician's pre-scription. The prescription NSAIDs are Motrin, a derivative of ibuprofen; Orudis and its sister brand Oruvail, a derivative of keto-profen; and Anaprox, a derivative of naproxen sodium. In Table 6.1, the NSAIDs that have been traditionally and commonly used for arthritis, both over-the-counter and prescription types, are dis-cussed as "traditional NSAIDs."

Over-the-Counter (OTC) NSAIDs
The non-prescription NSAIDs include all the salicylate group of drugs: aspirin, sold under the brand names Anacin, Bufferin, Excedrin, and many others; Aleve, a naproxen derivative; ibupro-fen and its brand-name derivatives, such as Motrin IB, Advil, and

Nuprin; and ketoprofen derivatives, found under the Actron and Orudis KT brand names. If you plan to take over-the-counter NSAIDs, speak to your physician or pharmacist first about their suitability for your condition and possible side effects.

COX-2 Inhibitors

A newer group of prescription NSAIDs that go by the name of COX-2 inhibitors appear to cause less stomach damage compared to other common NSAIDs, which have been traditionally pre-scribed. In recent years, two COX-2 inhibitors, rofecoxib (Vioxx) and valdecoxib (Bextra) have both been shown to increase the risk of heart attacks and strokes, and Bextra alone can result in a rare and life-threatening skin reaction. As a result, these two drugs have been withdrawn from the market. More recently, advisory groups in the United States and Canada have recommended that the Vioxx manufacturer (Merck) submit a new drug application to be reviewed and approved by the Food and Drug Administration (FDA) and Health Canada. No decision has been made regarding Bextra. However, Pfizer, its manufacturer, is discussing with the FDA the possibility of reinstating its use for patients who did well on the drug and suffered from fewer side effects.

Disease-Modifying, Anti-Rheumatic Drugs (DMARDs)

In the inflammatory forms of arthritis, such as rheumatoid arthri-tis, psoriatic arthritis, or lupus, joint damage is inevitable unless inflammation is controlled or the disease process is modified. DMARDs work by interfering with or suppressing the immune sys-tem so that it does not attack tissue. In this way, these drugs slow the progress of the disease. DMARDs are now prescribed in the early stages of disease and are usually quite effective. However, DMARDs can take time to show results, which is one reason why physicians prescribe these drugs early on in the disease process. Some DMARDs can take three to four months to take effect. Other drugs, such as NSAIDs or even corticosteroids, may be prescribed to help control the inflammation while the DMARDs are starting to work.

The DMARDs listed in Table 6.2 (beginning on the next page) are generally prescribed for patients with RA. However, some of these drugs are also prescribed for other conditions, such as juvenile chronic arthritis, ankylosing spondylitis, psoriatic arthritis, and lupus. Your physician will determine the dose you need, based on the disease you have, its severity, your age, your body weight, and any other medications you may be taking. With the exception of leflunomide and auranofin, all other DMARDs prescribed for inflammatory arthritis were developed originally to treat other diseases and medical conditions, such as malaria, cancer, and transplant rejection.

Because DMARDs suppress the immune system, consult your physician before getting any vaccinations while you are taking these drugs. If you are taking DMARDs, you should report any signs of infection, such as chills, fever, cough, or sore throat, to your physician.

Table 6.2
Disease-Modifying Anti-Rheumatic Drugs (DMARDs)

DISEASE-MODIFYING, ANTI-RHEUMATIC DRUGS, OR DMARDs

Uses/Effects	Side Effects	Monitoring
These are common arthritis medications. They relieve painful, swollen joints and slow joint damage. Several DMARDs may be used over the course of the disease. DMARDs take a few weeks or months to have an effect and may produce significant improvements for many patients. Exactly how they work is still unknown.	Side effects vary with each medicine. DMARDs may increase risk of infection, hair loss, and kidney or liver damage.	Physician monitoring allows the risk of toxicities to be weighed against the potential benefits.

AZATHIOPRINE (IMURAN)

Uses/Effects	Side Effects	Monitoring
This was first used in cancer chemotherapy and organ transplantation. It is used in patients who	Cough or hoarseness, fever or chills, loss of appetite, lower back or side pain, nausea or vomiting,	Before using this drug, tell your physician if you are taking allopurinal or have kidney or

Table 6.2
Disease-Modifying Anti-Rheumatic Drugs (DMARDs)
(*continued*)

AZATHIOPRINE (IMURAN)
(continued)

Uses/Effects	Side Effects	Monitoring
have not responded to other drugs and in combination therapy.	painful or difficult urination, unusual tiredness or weakness.	liver disease. This drug can reduce your ability to fight infection, so call your physician immediately if you develop chills, fever, or a cough. Regular blood and liver function tests are needed.

CYCLOSPORINE (NEORAL)

Uses/Effects	Side Effects	Monitoring
This medication was first used in organ transplantation to prevent rejection. It is used in patients who have not responded to other drugs.	Breathing, tender, or enlarged gums; high blood pressure; increased hair growth; trembling and shaking of hands.	Before taking this drug, tell your physician if you have one of the following: sensitivity to castor oil (if receiving the drug by injection), liver or kidney disease,

Table 6.2
Disease-Modifying Anti-Rheumatic Drugs (DMARDs)
(continued)

CYCLOSPORINE (NEORAL)
(continued)

Uses/Effects	Side Effects	Monitoring
		active infection, or high blood pressure. Using this drug may make you more susceptible to infection and certain cancers. Do not take live vaccines while on this drug.

HYDROXYCHLOROQUINE (PLAQUENIL IN THE UNITED STATES, AND APOHYDROXYQUINE IN CANADA)

Uses/Effects	Side Effects	Monitoring
It may take several months to notice the benefits of this drug, which include a reduction in the signs and symptoms of rheumatoid arthritis.	Diarrhea, eye problems (rare), headaches, loss of appetite, nausea or vomiting, stomach cramps or pain.	Physician monitoring is important, particularly if you have an allergy to any anti-malarial drug or a retinal abnormality.

Table 6.2
Disease-Modifying Anti-Rheumatic Drugs (DMARDs)
(continued)

GOLD THIOMALATE (MYOCHRYSINE)

Uses/Effects	Side Effects	Monitoring
This was one of the first DMARDs used to treat rheumatoid arthritis.	Redness or soreness of tongue; swelling or bleeding gums; skin rash or itching; ulcers or sores on lips, mouth, or throat; irritation on tongue. Joint pain may occur for one or two days after injection.	Before taking this drug, tell your physician if you have any of the following: lupus, skin rash, kidney disease, or colitis. Periodic urine and blood tests are needed to check for side effects.

LEFLUNOMIDE (ARAVA)

Uses/Effects	Side Effects	Monitoring
This drug reduces signs and symptoms and slows structural damage in joints caused by arthritis.	Bloody or cloudy urine; congestion in chest; cough; diarrhea; difficult, burning, or painful urination or breathing; fever; hair loss; headache; heartburn; loss of appetite; nausea	Before taking this medication, let your physician know if you have one of the following: active infection, liver disease, known immune deficiency, renal insufficiency, or underlying

Table 6.2
Disease-Modifying Anti-Rheumatic Drugs (DMARDs)
(continued)

LEFLUNOMIDE (ARAVA) (continued)

Uses/Effects	Side Effects	Monitoring
	and/or vomiting; skin rash; stomach pain; sneezing; and sore throat.	malignancy. You will need regular blood tests, including liver function tests. Leflunomide must not be taken during pregnancy because it may cause birth defects in humans.

METHOTREXATE (RHEUMATREX, TREXALL)

Uses/Effects	Side Effects	Monitoring
This drug can be taken by mouth or by injection and results in rapid improvement (it takes three to six weeks to begin working). It appears to be very effective, especially in combination with infliximab or etanercept. In general,	Abdominal discomfort, chest pain, chills, nausea, mouth sores, painful urination, sore throat, unusual tiredness or weakness.	Physician monitoring is important, particularly if you have an abnormal blood count, liver or lung disease, alcoholism, immune-system deficiency, or active infection. Methotrexate must

Table 6.2
Disease-Modifying Anti-Rheumatic Drugs (DMARDs)
(continued)

METHOTREXATE (RHEUMATREX, TREXALL) (continued)

Uses/Effects	Side Effects	Monitoring
it produces more favorable long-term responses than other DMARDs such as sulfasalazine, gold sodium thiomalate, and hydroxychloroquine.		not be taken during pregnancy because it may cause birth defects in humans.

SULFASALAZINE (AZULFIDINE IN THE UNITED STATES; SALAZOPYRIN IN CANADA)

Uses/Effects	Side Effects	Monitoring
This drug works to reduce the signs and symptoms of rheumatoid arthritis by suppressing the immune system.	Abdominal pain, aching joints, diarrhea, headache, sensitivity to sunlight, loss of appetite, nausea or vomiting, skin rash.	Physician monitoring is important, particularly if you are allergic to sulfa drugs or aspirin, or if you have a kidney, liver, or blood disease.

Biologic Response Modifiers (BRMs)

BRMs act by reducing the effects of cytokines, proteins that can cause joint inflammation. Like DMARDs, BRMs stop disease progression via immune-response suppression. In some cases, BRMs can produce a long-lasting disease remission. Because they are costly and have numerous side effects, they are generally only prescribed for patients who have failed to respond to other drugs. All BRMs increase the patient's risk of infection and a type of cancer called lymphoma. Another downside to these drugs is that they must be injected or given intravenously. They are sometimes administered together with standard DMARDs, such as methotrexate, in order to enhance the effect. Please see Table 6.3 for more detailed information about BRMs.

Table 6.3
Biologic Response Modifiers (BRMs)

BIOLOGIC RESPONSE MODIFIERS OR BRMs

Uses/Effects	Side Effects	Monitoring
These drugs selectively block parts of the immune system called cytokines. Cytokines play a role in inflammation. Long-term efficacy and safety of BRMs is uncertain.	Increased risk of infection, especially tuberculosis. Increased risk of pneumonia, and listeriosis (a food-borne illness caused by the bacterium *Listeria monocytogenes*).	It is important to avoid eating uncooked foods (including unpasteurized cheeses, cold cuts, and hot dogs) because undercooked food can cause listeriosis in patients taking biologic response modifiers.

TUMOR NECROSIS FACTOR INHIBITORS ETANERCEPT (ENBREL), INFLIXIMAB (REMICADE), ADALIMUMAB (HUMIRA)

Uses/Effects	Side Effects	Monitoring
These medications are highly effective for treating patients with an inadequate response to DMARDs. They may be prescribed in combination with some DMARDs, particularly	Etanercept: Pain or burning in throat; redness, itching, pain, and/or swelling at injection site; runny or stuffy nose. Infliximab: Abdominal pain, cough, dizziness,	Long-term efficacy and safety are uncertain. Physician monitoring is important, particularly if you have an active infection, exposure

Table 6.3
Biologic Response Modifiers (BRMs)
(continued)

TUMOR NECROSIS FACTOR INHIBITORS ETANERCEPT (ENBREL), INFLIXIMAB (REMICADE), ADALIMUMAB (HUMIRA) (continued)

Uses/Effects	Side Effects	Monitoring
methotrexate. Etanercept requires subcutaneous (beneath the skin) injections two times per week. Infliximab is taken intravenously (IV) during a two-hour procedure. It is administered with methotrexate. Adalimumab requires injection every two weeks. Long-term efficacy and safety are uncertain.	fainting, headache, muscle pain, runny nose, shortness of breath, sore throat, vomiting, wheezing. Adalimumab: Redness, rash, swelling, itching, bruising, sinus infection, headache, nausea.	to tuberculosis, or a central nervous system disorder. Evaluation for tuberculosis is necessary before treatment begins.

INTERLEUKIN-1 INHIBITOR ANAKINRA (KINERET)

Uses/Effects	Side Effects	Monitoring
This medication requires daily injections. Long-term efficacy and safety are uncertain.	Redness, swelling, bruising, or pain at the injection site; headache; upset stomach; diarrhea; runny nose; stomach pain.	Physician monitoring is required.

Table 6.3
Biologic Response Modifiers (BRMs)
(continued)

MONOCLONAL ANTIBODY RITUXIMAB (RITUXAN)

Uses/Effects	Side Effects	Monitoring
This medication is given intravenously every two weeks. An intravenous dose of steroid is usually given prior to the medication to reduce side effects.	Abdominal pain, nausea, vomiting, diarrhea; headache, back pain, or aching joints; rash or flushing.	Periodic blood tests to check blood counts and follow disease activity. Discuss vaccinations with your physician and advise your physician of any scheduled surgeries.

TI-CELL COSTIMULATION MODULATOR ABATACEPT (ORENCIA)

Uses/Effects	Side Effects	Monitoring
Abatacept is given by intravenous infusion once per month.	Nausea and diarrhea; headache and dizziness; back pain or aching joints; rash or flushing.	Periodic blood tests to check blood counts and monitor disease activity. Discuss vaccinations with your physician and advise your physician of any planned surgies.

Corticosteroids

Corticosteroids are among the most effective and oldest drugs used to treat inflammation. They must be administered sparingly and in low doses. High doses can cause brittle bones or osteoporosis, high blood pressure, cataracts, and numerous other side effects. Corticosteroid dosage can be effective, even when it is limited, if the drug is used in conjunction with DMARDs such as methotrexate. Corticosteroids are listed in Table 6.4.

Corticosteroid injections into an inflamed joint, a tendon sheath, or bursa can quickly reduce pain and inflammation. These injections are administered when one joint or a few joints are not responding to oral medication in the early stages of the disease. The benefit can last several months, provided the joint is rested for a few days after the injection. Tendon sheaths and bursae are also lined with synovial tissue; therefore, if this tissue becomes inflamed, injections can be very effective in reducing the inflammation. Injections can be repeated but not continuously and not frequently, as this can aggravate an already diseased joint.

Table 6.4
Corticosteroids

CORTICOSTEROIDS

Uses/Effects	Side Effects	Monitoring
Steroids are given by mouth or injection. They are used to relieve inflammation and reduce swelling.	Increased appetite, indigestion, nervousness, or restlessness.	For all corticosteroids, let your physician know if you have one of the following: fungal infection, history of tuberculosis, underactive thyroid, herpes simplex of the eye, high blood pressure, osteoporosis, or stomach ulcer.

METHYLPREDNISOLONE (MEDROL)

Uses/Effects	Side Effects	Monitoring
Available in pill form or an injection in a joint. Improvements are seen in several hours up to twenty-four hours after administration. There is potential for serious side effects, especially at high doses. They are used for severe flares and when the disease does not respond to NSAIDs or DMARDs.	Osteoporosis, mood changes, fragile skin, easy bruising, fluid retention, weight gain, muscle weakness, onset or worsening of diabetes, cataracts, increased risk of infection, high blood pressure.	Physician monitoring for continued effectiveness of medication and for side effects is needed.

Viscosupplement Drugs

Other medications that can be injected into joints to treat osteoarthritis are Synvisc, Neovisc, and Orthovisc; these drugs are referred to as viscosupplement drugs. They consist of thick (viscous) fluid that is made from a substance called hyaluronan found in normal joint synovial fluid. The viscosupplement drugs improve the natural viscosity and elasticity of synovial fluid and act as shock absorbers and joint lubricants, improving joint function. Administering viscosupplement drugs is comparable to putting oil on a rusty hinge. Viscosupplement drugs are not listed in the tables in Chapter 6.

Drugs Used to Treat Fibromyalgia

Although no single drug has been developed or approved to treat fibromyalgia, off-label prescribing by physicians is quite common in managing this disease. In the past, it was not unheard of for a physician to prescribe corticosteroids to treat fibromyalgia to their patient's detriment, in the mistaken belief that they were treating rheumatoid arthritis. This practice is uncommon these days.

A number of medications developed to treat other conditions have been effective in treating fibromyalgia. These include antidepressants such as amitriptyline (Endrep); muscle relaxants such as cyclobenzaprine (Cycloflex or Flexeril); certain analgesics, including the powerful tramadol (Ultram or Ultracet); and drugs used to treat anxiety, such as fluoxetine (Prozac). Research is underway in Germany to determine the effects of a promising new drug on pain perception in patients with fibromyalgia. This drug, Namenda (memantine HCL), has been shown to dampen activity in those areas of the brain that are responsible for the processing of pain and are hyperactive in fibromyalgia patients.

Table 6.5
Medications Used to Treat Fibromyalgia

CYCLOBENZAPRINE (CYCOFLEX, FLEXERIL)

Uses/Effects	Side Effects	Monitoring
Muscle relaxant.	Blurred vision; dizziness; light-headedness; drowsiness; dry mouth.	Do not use with alcohol; antihistamines; tranquilizers; sleeping medications; narcotic pain medication. Physician monitoring for effectiveness and side effects is needed.

DULOXETINE (CYMBALTA) AND FLUOXETINE (PROZAC)

Uses/Effects	Side Effects	Monitoring
Antidepressant	Anxiety or nervousnes; decrease in appetite and sexual desire; diarrhea or constipation; dry mouth; headache; hives or itching; sweating; skin rash; trembling or shaking; nausea; trouble sleeping.	Do not use with alcohol; antihistamines; narcotics; dental anesthetics; aspirin or NSAIDs. Watch for agitation and suicidal tendencies. Physician monitoring is needed.

Table 6.5
Medications Used to Treat Fibromyalgia
(continued)

AMITRIPTYLINE HYDROCHLORIDE (ENDEP)

Uses/Effects	Side Effects	Monitoring
Antidepressant	Constipation; dizziness; tiredness; headache; dry mouth; drowsiness; weight gain.	Do not use with other anti-depressants. Inform physician if you have a history of seizures, urinary retention, glaucoma, heart problems, or chronic eye problems. Physician monitoring is needed.

TRAMADOL (ULTRAM OR ULTRACET)

Uses/Effects	Side Effects	Monitoring
Analgesic	Dizziness; drowsiness; constipation or diarrhea; nausea, loss of appetite; sweating.	Do not drive or operate heavy machinery until you know how your body reacts to this medication; do not stop medication abruptly or increase dose on your own. Physician monitoring is needed.

Drugs Used to Treat Gout

Gout is one of the few rheumatic illnesses that can be treated easily. Drugs used to treat gout fall into two main categories: those that quickly reduce pain and inflammation, and those that reduce future attacks. NSAIDs, corticosteroids, or colchicine (a specific anti-inflammatory medication for gout) are used in the early stages of gout to treat inflammation and pain. If the cause of gout is the body producing too much uric acid or not excreting uric acid properly, then allopurinol (Lopurin or Zyloprim) is used to slow uric-acid production. Ingestion of uric-acid-lowering medications is lifelong and can dramatically reduce future and painful attacks of gout. See Table 6.6, starting on the next page.

Table 6.6
Medications Used to Treat Gout

COLCHICINE (AVAILABLE ONLY AS GENERIC)

Uses/Effects	Side Effects	Monitoring
Reduce inflammation	Diarrhea; nausea or vomiting; stomach pain; neuropathy (any disease of the nerves).	Do not use if you have kidney, liver, or intestinal disease; ongoing infection; or if you are taking immunosuppressive drugs. Physician monitoring is needed.

PROBENECID (BENEMID, PROBALAN)

Uses/Effects	Side Effects	Monitoring
To help kidneys excrete uric acid.	Nausea or vomiting; loss of appetite; headache.	Physician monitoring is needed as it is a lifelong medication.

ALLOPURINOL (LOPURIN, ZYLOPRIM)

Uses/Effects	Side Effects	Monitoring
To help kidneys excrete uric acid.	Itching; hives; skin rash.	Do not use if you are on azathioprine (Imuran) or if you have kidney disease. Do not start or stop allopurinol during a flare of gout. Physician monitoring is needed.

Looking Forward

This chapter covers the use of traditional prescription and certain over-the-counter drugs usually recommended by physicians to treat arthritis and related disorders. The following chapter addresses pain management for arthritis and features information on other proven ways to deal with arthritis pain in addition to medication use. Herbal remedies, multi-vitamin ingestion, and other non-traditional remedies such as cobra venom and bee stings will be covered in Chapter 18.

Chapter 7

How Can I Manage My Arthritis Pain?

Pain in joints and muscles is one of the most common reasons for people to visit their doctor (second only to upper-respiratory infections). In this chapter, we will address a topic that is foremost in the minds of many arthritis patients. Pain can have a major impact on a person's ability to carry out daily activities and to enjoy an independent lifestyle. It can be invisible to others and is often not well understood.

The ways in which individuals manage pain or seek relief are too numerous to list. In their search for relief, people can spend great amounts of time and money trying an endless variety of "cures" and pain-relieving products, which may or may not be helpful. This chapter will provide an explanation of the causes of pain in arthritis and some background on the factors that can contribute to pain. In this chapter, we also share several pain-relieving strategies. The information here is based on scientific research and is designed to help you choose pain-management techniques that have been proven to be useful and practical. Most importantly, this chapter is intended to help you to stay positive and active, and to take the steps you need to control your pain so that it does not control you or your life.

**A well informed patient is better
able to manage pain.**

Strong research indicates that a patient's thoughts, feelings, emotions, and behavior, as well as the attitudes and responses of his or her family, can influence the experience of pain from arthritis. Research has also shown that patients who are well informed about their condition, how joints work, and the reasons for the pain have a better sense of control over the pain, are more self-confident, and are better able to adjust their daily activities to their symptoms. This has led experts to recommend that patient and family education be a central part of a pain-management program. The more you know about pain, the more prepared you are to manage it successfully.

WHAT IS PAIN?

The International Association for the Study of Pain defines pain as "an unpleasant sensory and emotional experience associated with actual or potential tissue damage, or described in terms of such damage." Pain is a subjective experience that individuals learn about throughout life; perceptions of pain are based on early experiences. Pain is an unpleasant experience, but it does have a purpose, which is to protect us. It is pain that makes us pull a hand away from a hot surface or a sharp object. It is clear that pain can shield us from harm. What is not so clear is exactly how it works.

All sensations that we experience result from the workings of the nervous system. The human nervous system is more complex than the most sophisticated electronic wiring. The ancient Greeks first described and analyzed our wire-like nerves, which carry sensations from virtually everywhere in the body to the brain. Then, in 1664, the French scientist Rene Descartes suggested that pain travels on a single, simple pathway from the skin of the extremities to the spinal cord, the brain, and then back again to the source of the pain. He suggested that pain was an alarm signal designed to indicate harm. From that basic understanding, scientists have worked for centuries to learn more about this astonishingly complex network that touches and controls almost every part of the human body. Figure 7.1 is a very basic illustration of Descartes's concept.

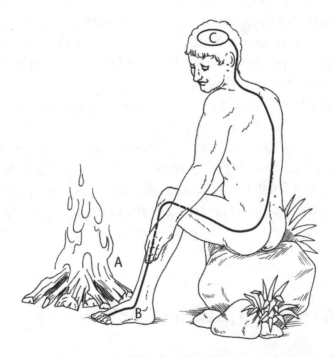

Figure 7.1
*Descartes described the pain system as a simple, single pathway
from the skin to the brain.*

In 1965, Canadian psychologist Ronald Melzack and his colleague, Patrick Wall, introduced what is known as the gate-control theory, which proposed that the pain pathway is more complex than Descartes's original concept. The gate-control theory states that signals from the skin travel to the spinal cord, where a mechanism acts as a kind of gate, shutting down or opening up and thus controlling the flow of sensations. The gate opens, closes, or partially closes depending on what kinds of signals it receives from the brain—emotions, memories, or even cultural attitudes.

Scientists now know that the spinal cord serves a number of different purposes in relaying signals to the brain and transmitting messages from the brain to the extremities. Our current understanding of the gate-control theory guides modern medical pain-control strategies, influencing how medications and physical and behavioral measures are employed in the effort to allay pain.

Current research on the nervous system indicates that our nerve cells are grouped in bundles like the fibers of a rope and may be very short or run the full length of the body. Some nerve fibers, called afferent fibers, carry sensations, such as pain, *to* the spinal cord and brain. Efferent fibers deliver messages *away* from the brain and spinal cord, carrying command signals to muscles to contract in order to move the body part away from the harm. The signals may also travel to body organs, such as the stomach, to release digestive enzymes. Figure 7.2 (on the next page) shows the response of the nervous system when an injury occurs, in this case a stubbed toe.

WHAT IS CAUSING MY PAIN?

There are many possible causes of pain. Therefore, the first step in finding out why you hurt should be a complete assessment by a qualified health-care professional who can help determine the

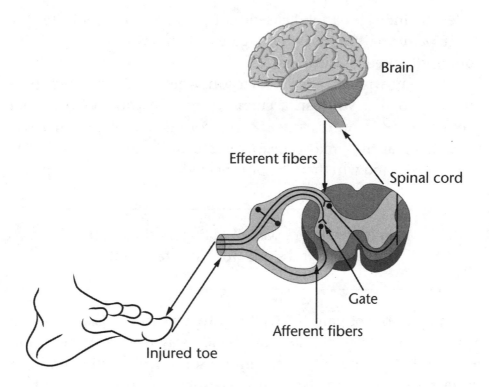

Brain

Efferent fibers

Spinal cord

Gate

Afferent fibers

Injured toe

Figure 7.2
Afferent fibers carry signals to the brain.
Efferent fibers carry messages from the brain.
The gate controls the flow of sensations.

cause of your pain. You also need to know which type of arthritis you have, because that will influence your pain treatment.

When you visit your health-care provider, be prepared to describe your pain, its intensity, and its location, and be able to explain what makes the pain better or worse. It is helpful if you can describe the quality of the pain in simple terms, such as burning, aching, stabbing, or throbbing, as well as whether it is constant or variable. There are many pain scales to help you determine how bad your pain typically is. Commonly, on the visual analogue scale, "0" indicates a total absence of pain and "10" indicates the worst pain you can imagine. Figure 7.3 shows examples of two commonly used pain scales.

You may wish to make a diary in which you can track pain episodes so that you can accurately describe your pain to your physician. In a pain diary, you can record details about what you were doing at the time you experienced the pain, what you tried to relieve it, and whether or not it helped.

**Pain is our body's way of telling us something
is wrong! It is a signal for us to take action.**

The purpose of pain is to tell you that *something* is wrong. Just as pain can tell you to take your hand away from a flame, it can tell you that you need to rest, perform some activity differently, or protect an inflamed wrist by using a splint. Your pain diary may help you see a pattern or show you which things help you manage the pain and which things may make it seem worse.

Arthritis pain is caused by a number of factors:

✦ Inflammation—the process (described in Chapter 2) that causes the swelling and tenderness of the joints.

✦ Damage—to the joint surfaces or the tissues around the joints, which is due to injury, stress, or pressure on the joints.

✦ Fatigue—which can be part of the disease process itself or simply a result of becoming overtired. Fatigue can make your pain seem worse and more difficult to manage.

✦ Stress or depression—possibly caused by having limited movement and less ability to do things you enjoy.

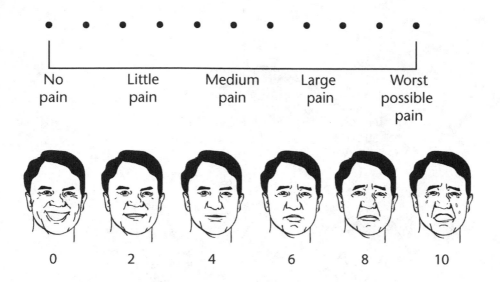

From Wong DL, Hockenberry-Eaton M, Wilson D, Winkelstein ML, Ahmann E, DiVito-Thomas PA: *Whaley and Wong's Nursing Care of Infants and Children,* ed. 6, St. Louis, 1999, Mosby, p. 1153.

Figure 7.3
Pain scales are used to describe pain intensity and to monitor response to treatment.

✦ Anxiety—triggered by worries about the future, lost time from work, and changes in relationships and lifestyle. These can all affect your ability to cope with pain, making pain seem worse.

✦ Focusing on the pain—when you allow pain to dominate your thoughts, pain can become more overwhelming and more difficult to treat.

When any of these factors is present, you can get caught in what is referred to as a "pain cycle." A pain cycle is illustrated in Figure 7.4.

THE PAIN CYCLE

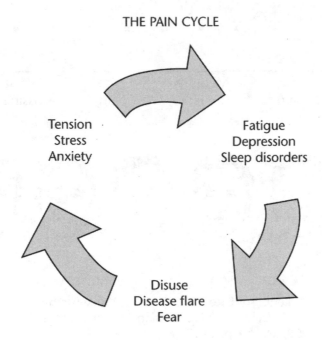

Tension
Stress
Anxiety

Fatigue
Depression
Sleep disorders

Disuse
Disease flare
Fear

Figure 7.4
Negative factors can add up to worsen pain and increase distress.

Some types of pain are easier to treat than others. Long-lasting pain, like arthritis pain, is more difficult to treat than pain resulting from a cut finger or a bruised shin. Pain that persists for more than three months is referred to as chronic pain. Learning to manage chronic pain can be the hardest part of having arthritis, but you can learn to manage it by thinking of pain as a signal to take positive action rather than thinking of it as an ordeal you have to endure. A positive attitude and active participation in your treatment plan will put you in control and help you break the cycle of pain.

**The keys to successful pain management are a
positive attitude and active participation
in the treatment plan.**

HOW CAN I BREAK THE PAIN CYCLE?

Dr. Melzack's gate-control theory ties into the concept of the pain cycle. After more than twenty years, researchers have learned that when harm or pain signals are traveling to the spinal cord, these signals can be altered by other sensory messages. These so-called counter-messages, such as painkillers, heat, cold, electrical stimulation, relaxation, or distraction, can close the gate so that pain sensations do not reach the brain, offering some relief .

The chemicals that your body produces to block pain signals are called *endorphins*. Endorphins are naturally occurring, morphine-like, painkilling substances that can decrease the pain sensation. They are produced in response to external factors such as medication, exercise, hot or cold applications, excitement, or distraction. Endorphins are good things, and they can close the gate.

You can break the pain cycle by understanding what may be causing or contributing to the pain and stopping the pain before it starts or worsens. The key is to take control of pain before it takes control of you. There is no single method of pain management that is always effective for everyone, but with some concerted effort, each person can learn the techniques that are most often effective for him or herself. To do so, you need to be a creative problem solver and get ahead of the pain. For example, if your joints are swollen and tender, taking pain-relieving or anti-inflammatory medications may help. Applying ice or resting the swollen joints may also bring relief. If a joint is damaged by arthritis, you may need to support that joint by using a brace, by adapting your activities, or by avoiding situations that place more stress on that joint.

**You can learn to close the pain gate
and break the pain cycle.**

Fatigue is often a part of having a chronic disease. It can also be the result of having to spend more of your available energy, or due to the fact that simple tasks may be more difficult as a result of pain or stiffness. Think of yourself as having a cup full of energy to last your whole day. If you spend three quarters of that cup of energy adapting to the limitations imposed by your arthritis, you will not have enough energy left over to do things that are enjoyable and worthwhile. In this case, you may become tired, the gate will open, and you will experience more pain.

WHAT ROLE DO EMOTIONS PLAY IN PAIN MANAGEMENT?

Your mind and feelings play an important role in how you experience pain and how you react or adjust to illness. Feelings of depression or helplessness can lead to decreased activity, low self-esteem, and increased pain.

Just as it benefits you to manage your energy expenditure, you can help to control your pain by managing your stress levels. If you are aware that you are going through a stressful period in your life, which may be creating tension or causing you to lose sleep, finding ways to relieve the stress, or turning your attention to positive action, can help prevent your pain from increasing. Techniques such as relaxation or visualization can make a difference in your life.

Maintaining a positive attitude and adjusting your thoughts and actions will help you to stay in control of your life. Try to focus on wellness, not sickness. Think of the things that you *can* do rather than listing those you can't. Maintain a sense of humor; laughter releases endorphins! Researchers in Japan have recently reported that certain chemicals related to inflammation within the body were significantly affected for the better following laughter.

**Control your pain by managing
your energy and stress levels.**

Keep your family ties and your friendships strong. Research shows that people whose lives are affected by pain are better able to cope and are less depressed and less disabled when they have a supportive social network. Friends and loving partners can help you beat depression, distract you from pain, and help you when you need support. Chapter 14 can help you learn more about the emotional issues relating to arthritis and pain, and Chapter 15 has more information about maintaining closeness in intimate relationships, which have been shown to be critical to pain-management success.

Avoid focusing on pain. The time you spend thinking about pain can increase your tension and discomfort. Pain is reported to be worse for people who focus on pain than for those who do not. Doing something that is easy and pleasurable can improve your mood. If you cannot ignore the pain, it can help to think of it in a different way, perhaps as a message from your body to change position, elevate your legs, or take a short walk.

Avoiding Pain Behaviors

Pain behaviors send signals to the world around you that you are in pain and need help. Examples of pain behaviors are:

✦ Limping.

✦ Holding an arm tightly against the body.

✦ Holding onto walls or furniture when walking.

✦ Grimacing or wincing.

✦ Sighing.

✦ Moaning.

✦ Acting listless.

When you are first experiencing pain, these behaviors are understandable. But if you really think about it, you will realize that doing things like making faces, holding onto furniture, and moaning and complaining do not actually relieve your pain. In fact, the tension produced by these behaviors has been shown to increase pain. By controlling your pain behaviors, you can present a more positive aspect to friends and family and to yourself!

Self-Talk

It is easy when you are experiencing pain and feeling depressed to sink down into negative thoughts and "self-talk." Negative self-talk can cause you to see yourself as injured or disabled. For better or for worse, self-talk influences how you look at life and how you behave.

For example, one morning, instead of saying, "I don't want to go out today— it's too much trouble and it might rain," try saying, "It looks like rain, but I always feel better after I exercise. I'll just take my umbrella and see what happens." If you listen to yourself and follow your own excellent advice, you are a lot more likely to get moving. Who knows? Perhaps the sun will even come out, and by leaving the house, you will have put yourself in a position to run into a neighbor whose company you enjoy. In this example, by starting the day with some positive self-talk, you distract yourself, gain the benefit of some exercise, and enjoy yourself in the process.

Changing from a negative outlook to a positive one can be a challenge. Table 7.1 will help get you started. Practicing positive self-talk may feel a little strange at first, but you'll soon discover what a difference it can make to you and to others around you.

Table 7.1
Negative Versus Positive Self-Talk

NEGATIVE SELF-TALK	POSITIVE SELF-TALK
The pain is the same. I'll never get any better.	The healing process takes time. Even though it's slow, I know I am making some progress.
I don't think these medications are going to help.	I believe that these medications will help me, but the doctor told me that they are slow-acting, so I need to be patient.
I don't think I can manage to work at all.	Even if I can't work full-time anymore, I can try to work part-time.
I can't go on social outings; I'm in too much pain.	Even though I'm in pain, if I rest before I go out, perhaps I will have the energy to enjoy myself. Maybe being around other people will take my mind off of my pain.

Relaxation Techniques

When you have arthritis and are in pain, you experience both physical and emotional stress. Pain and stress affect the body in similar ways by making your muscles tighten, your breathing shallow and rapid, and your heart rate to increase and your blood pressure to rise. Relaxation is useful in dealing with these effects and makes it easier to deal with pain. Learning to calm and control your mind and body is not always easy, and you may need to try several methods to find the best way to relax both the mind and body.

Some relaxation techniques you may want to try include the following:

✦ Relaxation audiotapes can guide you through the gradual relaxation techniques.

✦ Gentle yoga or tai chi classes can teach you to employ slow, rhythmic motions to calm your body and mind.

✦ Guided imagery is a technique in which you train your mind to focus on pleasant images.

✦ Prayer or meditation is very relaxing and comforting to some people.

You may need to work with an instructor to get relaxation methods underway, but after a while, you'll be able to take over these techniques and use them when and where you need them.

Learning to relax is a good investment.

You can seek assistance in learning to relax, refocus, and adjust to your changing lifestyle and habits as well as to the emotional impact of your disease by discussing your feelings and fears with a social worker or by joining a support group or an exercise group, such as a pool program in warm water.

Finding Positive Ways to Deal with the Pain

When dealing with chronic pain, it is easy to fall into unhealthy habits or practices, such as taking more medicine than was prescribed or drinking alcohol to escape pain. If you are using up medication faster than usual, spending an excessive amount of time in bed, using alcohol for pain relief, or talking about pain a good deal, you need to consider some new ways to handle the pain.

If you are slipping into unhealthy habits, discuss this with your doctor, nurse, or other professional who is familiar with pain management, and ask about other ways to manage pain. Arthritis and the accompanying pain can be overwhelming at times. Don't hesitate to seek out the resources you need to help you stay in control.

Changing your habits and finding new ways to deal with your pain will help you feel better. You can do this by replacing an old, unhealthy habit with something positive. Reward yourself each time you make a positive change in your habits, behaviors, or attitudes. Get a massage, take a warm bath, relax with soothing music, or make the time to phone a friend.

THE PHYSICAL MANAGEMENT OF PAIN

In conjunction with maintaining a positive approach to your illness, there are many things that you can do physically to help control your pain, and there are many people who can help you.

As the key player on your health-care team, you have the responsibility to become a "pain manager" and to explore the many options available to help you. The following suggestions are intended to help you stay physically active and to relieve your pain.

Medical Pain Management

Once you have an accurate diagnosis and understand the reasons for your pain, you will want to develop a management plan for controlling your pain. You should work with your doctor and other members of your health-care team to determine which strategies are likely to be most successful in your personal situation. Chapter 6 contains extensive information about a variety of medications and drug therapies. Please refer to it for specifics about the different types of recommended medications.

Joint inflammation produces pain. Therefore, if you have inflammatory arthritis, inflammation control will be the main aim of the pain-management plan. This step must be undertaken to provide a foundation for any other treatments you may choose. Chapter 6 explains the relationship between anti-inflammatory medications and pain-relieving medications.

Your pharmacist or your physician can help you get the maximum benefit from your medications. If you have inflammatory arthritis, it may be that your disease is very active and you might need to increase or change the medication in order to reduce the inflammation that is ultimately causing your pain. A pharmacist or a physician can also help you time your pain-medication dosages so that their effects are at their maximum when you need them the most.

Take your medications exactly as they are prescribed, and be sure that you understand the action of the drug and its potential side effects by discussing them with your doctor or your pharmacist.

Some arthritis drugs take a few weeks to become effective, so don't discontinue them because you feel they are not working without first consulting your doctor or pharmacist. Remember—this is a team approach.

If you have one or two persistently painful joints that don't seem to be responding to pain medication, your doctor may suggest an injection of cortisone directly into the joint to control the inflammation. These injections usually reduce the swelling and pain, and the benefits can last a few weeks or several months, allowing you to stay active and continue your exercise program. You will likely be advised to rest the joint for a few days after the injection to allow the medication to work more effectively. If you have osteoarthritis, three to five weekly injections of viscosupplement drugs can provide relief by improving the quality of the synovial fluid in the joint. These injections are costly, but they are an option you may want to discuss with your doctor. You can read more about viscosupplements and corticosteroids in Chapter 6.

If you are having joint pain at rest that is not responding to medications and is disturbing your sleep or making it impossible for you to perform your usual activities, surgery may be indicated. Your doctor is the best person to tell you if surgery is an option for you, and he or she can also make a referral to an orthopedic surgeon if that step is warranted. See Chapter 17 for more discussion of this topic.

Talk with your doctor about any other treatment plans you may be considering, including naturopathic treatments or herbal remedies, and ask about the safety and effectiveness of these as well as possible interactions with medications. Chapter 18 discusses these choices in detail.

Visit your doctor to begin a treatment plan, learn about pain management, or get referrals.

A wide range of approaches are available to you to help you control your pain. Before making your treatment choices, seek the advice of your professional health-care team. Your doctor can advise you about pain mananagement and make referrals to other health-care providers, such as physical or occupational therapists or social workers who can also help you. Your physician may also be aware of community resources such as support groups or pool programs. Be sure that your treatment team members communicate with you and with the other providers whom you choose to be part of the team. Chapter 4 can help you better understand the roles and expertise areas of the various health-care team members.

Electrical Devices or Modalities

In addition to medications, a variety of electrical devices or modalities may be used in clinics or rehabilitation facilities to treat painful conditions such as arthritis. Some are appropriate for home use by patients, but most require regular visits to a clinical facility, and this can be expensive and time consuming. Table 7.2 on the next page outlines the most common modalities and their effects, provides some comments regarding their practicality for home use, and briefly lists research supporting their efficacy. For more information on some of these treatments, see Chapter 18. Ask your doctor or physiotherapist about which, if any, of these may be best for you.

Proven Home Remedies

Pain management does not have to be "alternative" or "high-tech" to be effective. There are several strategies for pain relief that you can easily try in the comfort and privacy of your own home.

Table 7.2
Common Electrical Devices or Modalities
Used to Treat Arthritis Pain

MODALITY	EFFECT	COMMENTS
Ultrasound	Sound waves administered through an applicator provide deep heat to the tissues.	Limited research evidence for its utility, although it has been shown to reduce joint tenderness. Not suitable for home use.
Trancutaneous Electrical Nerve Stimulation (TENS)	Electrodes, applied to the skin, interfere with pain signals, closing the gate. The current stimulates the release of endorphins.	Some studies have shown TENS to relieve pain for three or more hours, improve sleep, and reduce the pain signals. More research is needed. Portable units can be suitable for home use. This treatment can be time-consuming if applied to more than two sites.
Low-Level Laser	A light source that generates extremely pure light and causes reactions in the cells.	Studies on its effects (on the hands of patients with RA and OA) show conflicting results, but some studies report short-term reduction in pain and morning stiffness. Not suitable for home use.
Acupuncture	The insertion of thin needles to specific points	This is a widely used treatment by many practitioners, but the studies

MODALITY	EFFECT	COMMENTS
Acupuncture (continued)	on the body stimulates release of endorphins. May be combined with electrical current.	so far have provided no strong evidence to support its use. Not suitable for home use, although small, handheld devices are available for individuals to use on their own.

Using applications of ice or heat can provide relief of pain and stiffness in muscles and joints. The simplest forms, such as a bag of frozen vegetables wrapped in a moist towel or a damp, smoothly folded towel in a plastic bag and heated in the microwave for one minute, are just as effective as costly commercial products. You should have at least one layer of moist toweling between the heat or ice and your skin to help spread the effect evenly and to prevent burns. A ten- to fifteen-minute treatment is advised, as a longer period may overheat or cool the tissues and cause damage to the skin.

Some precautions are advised when considering the application of heat or cold. Never apply heat or ice on top of analgesic creams or ointments. Do not lie or rest a limb on top of a heat or ice pack, because the weight of your limb compresses the insulating layer of toweling, bringing your skin closer to the source of heat or cold. This can cause the skin to burn. In inflammatory arthritis, alternating heat with cold is not advised, because heat and cold have opposite effects on your circulation. If you have circulatory problems or color changes in your hands or feet on exposure to cold, avoid the use of cold and discuss the use of heat with your health-care provider.

Cold is thought to "close the gate," to control pain and muscle spasm, and to be best for use on actively inflamed joints. Heat, on the other hand, increases nerve conduction and can increase pain if it is applied to inflamed joints. Heat should not be applied if joints are warm and swollen. For mildly inflamed joints, however, heat can relieve stiffness or the "gel" phenomenon (the thickening of the lubricating fluid within the joint that tends to occur during periods of rest). Heat can also reduce pain in the tissues surrounding the joint, muscle spasm, and the stiffness of joints affected by osteoarthritis.

A form of heat treatment that has been shown to reduce pain and stiffness in the hands involves the application of heated paraffin wax. The hands are dipped in heated wax eight to ten times, put into plastic bags, and wrapped in towels for about fifteen minutes. The process is cumbersome, as it is difficult to do both hands at one time and heating the wax can be problematic. However, there are thermostatically controlled wax baths available for home use. A far simpler and equally effective treatment is to apply oil (massage oil, baby oil, olive oil, or salad oil) liberally to the hands, then put on ordinary rubber dishwashing gloves and exercise your hands in a hot-water-filled sink or tub. Less risk, less mess, and completely portable! When combined with simple hand exercises, it relieves pain and morning stiffness.

Here are several other simple ideas that you can use to try to manage your pain at home:

✦ Try changing positions by standing up and moving around, or bend and stretch your joints a few times.

✦ Balance rest with activity. Rest has been shown to reduce pain and swelling when your arthritis is very active, so you may need to cut back and do a little less until the inflammation is under control. Resume activities gradually.

✦ Support painful, inflamed joints by using your splints or resting your joints in a position of comfort.

✦ Use good posture in whatever you may be doing: sitting, standing, or walking. Ask a health professional to show you the correct posture.

✦ Analgesic (pain-relieving) rubs or ointments can provide temporary relief. Some contain anti-inflammatory ingredients, which are absorbed into your body. Ask your pharmacist for advice before using any medications. Do not use analgesics with hot or cold packs, and do not apply an analgesic before putting on splints or other supports.

✦ Think of easier ways to do things. Make use of devices, canes, utensils with padded handles, and raised seating. Chapter 13 covers these topics in more detail.

Exercise, Exercise, Exercise!

The benefits of exercise for people with arthritis have been proven in studies time and time again. Exercise is probably the single most effective thing that you can do to control your pain and to stay involved in everyday activities. By exercising safely, you keep your bones, joints, and muscles healthy. Strong muscles help to protect your joints.

Exercising regularly can:

✦ Decrease the symptoms of arthritis and reduce pain.

✦ Improve your sense of well-being.

✦ Increase your activity tolerance.

✦ Improve your mobility.

✦ Help with weight control.

Please refer to Chapters 9, 10, 11, and 12 for more details about the best types of exercises for you.

There are three different types of exercise that have been proven repeatedly to benefit arthritis patients. You should exercise to strengthen large muscles, to increase your joint mobility, and to increase your aerobic capacity or fitness level. All of these types of exercise can relieve your pain.

Do a combination of these three types of exercises for a total of at least thirty minutes, several times per week. This may sound difficult and time-consuming if you have never exercised or have exercised very little, but this is not difficult if you break it down into just ten minutes of exercise three times a day. You can choose where and when to get your exercise, and you can exercise alone or in a group. You can walk or cycle with a friend, you can dance, or you can go to a warm-water exercise program. If you choose, you can enjoy a social activity at the same time.

Take it easy at the beginning, particularly if you have not exercised in the past. Many people with arthritis become deconditioned as a result of being inactive for long periods of time. Talk to your health-care provider before undertaking an exercise program if you have heart problems, high blood pressure, or dizziness. "Start slow and go low!" is sound advice for beginners. Start your exercise regime slowly, with low intensity and few repetitions. As you build confidence and tolerance, you will be able to speed up and do more repetitions.

Set moderate beginning goals for your exercise program, such as, "I want to be able to walk six blocks within three weeks." To begin, try walking two blocks, remembering that you have to walk back. Remember to wear comfortable, supportive shoes. If, after progressing to a total of four blocks, you experience more than two hours of increased joint discomfort or pain, it may be that your limit is two or three blocks. This is known as the "two-hour pain rule." You can apply this rule to any physical activity you choose to try. If you feel more than two hours of pain, cut back, then work back up to four blocks once you can walk two or three blocks without any ill effects.

A physiotherapist can help you begin your exercise program if you have severe arthritis, have had problems exercising in the past, or have particular problems with one or two joints. The physiotherapist can also teach you to use heat or ice prior to exercising and again afterward.

**Set exercise goals, "go slow, go low," and
follow the two-hour pain rule.**

Explore the exercise opportunities in your community and have your progress monitored by your health-care team. You are the only person who can do your exercises! The health-care team is there to recommend the types of exercise suited to you, teach you how to do the exercises, and cheer you on as you achieve your exercise goals, but meeting those goals is entirely up to you.

The Arthritis Self-Management Program

The Arthritis Self-Management Program, a program available throughout Canada and the United States, has been shown to have a significantly positive effect on people who attend its six weekly sessions. The program is led by people with arthritis who have personally experienced the challenges the disease can offer. Members of the group offer encouragement, support, and problem solving, not only to the patient but also to family members. Check to see if a program is available near you. (See the resources section for further information.)

Looking Forward

Pain management is not easy, and it is difficult to go it alone. Make sure that you utilize the services your health-care team can provide. Managing your pain is key to leading a fulfilling life with arthritis, and it is well worth the effort you put into it. As you learn to manage your pain, don't forget to congratulate and reward yourself for accomplishing this important aspect of living with arthritis!

This chapter has provided an explanation of the ways in which pain affects people with arthritis and has offered suggestions to help you become an effective pain manager. Your health-care team and other resources, such as friends and family, can support you as you learn to manage this aspect of arthritis. The following chapter will suggest ways in which you can adopt a healthy approach to life with arthritis in order to delay or prevent the disability that it can cause.

Chapter 8

How Can I
Stay Well and
Prevent Disability?

If you have arthritis, you may say to yourself, "How can I be well when I have a chronic condition?" and "How is it possible for me to prevent disability?" But it *is* possible to have arthritis and *not* be disabled and *continue* to aspire to wellness. Even though, for the most part, you as an individual are not able to prevent the onset of arthritis, there are many things that you can do to lessen your chances of disability and to promote your own wellness in the bargain even when you are diagnosed with arthritis.

The first part of this chapter defines the terms "wellness" and "disability" and discusses the effects arthritis can have on various important aspects of your life in addition to your physical well-being. The last part of the chapter explains the difference between the terms "impairment" and "disability" and describes ways in which disability can be reduced or prevented. In the discussion on disability, two case studies of patients with similar types of arthri-

181

tis are compared to illustrate how differently arthritis can affect individuals depending on their lifestyles.

IS THERE A DIFFERENCE BETWEEN HEALTH AND WELLNESS?

Your understanding of health and wellness can significantly influence what you do to make yourself healthy or ill. The World Health Organization (WHO) defines health as "not only the absence of infirmity or disease, but also a state of physical, mental, and social well-being." Wellness, similarly, is more than just not being ill. It has a somewhat broader meaning than the term "health." The concept of wellness refers to "a level of physical and emotional harmony that affords maximum resistance to disease and supports a sustained joy of living." (Source: Epilepsy Ontario)

Wellness is more than just not being sick.

Wellness has also been defined as an active process of becoming aware of and making choices toward a more successful existence. This definition shifts the focus away from illness toward a view of health that emphasizes the whole person. To achieve this state of wellness, individuals must take responsibility for their own overall health. Some believe that a wellness approach to living provides protection against disease by enabling a person to draw on his or her inner resources or abilities to promote healing. Wellness is pursued by people who are interested in recovery from or coping with ill health or specific health conditions, and also by healthy people who are interested in maintaining their best possible health.

WHAT FACTORS CONTRIBUTE TO MY WELLNESS?

Some experts believe that we need to balance several overlapping elements in order to achieve wellness. Figure 8.1 illustrates the interrelated elements that influence your well-being. By focusing on improving these aspects of your life and by understanding how these factors relate to each other, you can strive to control your symptoms before they control you. In the following sections, we briefly address the interrelated factors that can contribute to wellness. Various chapters throughout the book, particularly in Part II, contain more detailed information on these topics, and throughout this section, we refer you to other chapters for more information where appropriate.

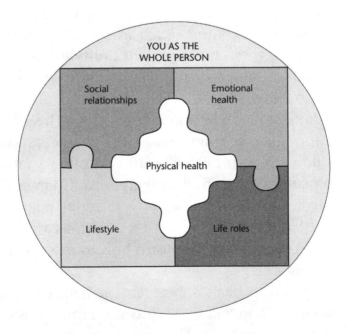

Figure 8.1
As a whole person, many factors affect your wellness.

Physical Health

If you have arthritis, it is natural that your attention will be direct-ed toward relieving physical symptoms and coping with the phys-ical effects of your condition. In fact, much of the information in this book is intended to help you get the most benefit out of the many physical treatment options that are available. However, it is important that while you are managing the physical effects of your diagnosis, you don't lose sight of the other important things that you can do to maintain or improve all aspects of your wellness (Figure 8.1). By remembering that you are more than just a body, you can position yourself to lead a rewarding and fulfilling life in spite of the challenges that having a condition such as arthritis can present. You may be a person with arthritis, but you do not have to be an "arthritic person."

Your physical health depends on many factors, some of which you cannot completely control—such as heredity, environment, gender, and age. But there are important lifestyle factors that you *can* control—such as diet, exercise, rest, attitude, and stress man-agement—as shown in Table 8.1.

Make good decisions about the aspects of your health that you can control, and take the time to read the chapters of this book that have to do with pain management and other strategies that can help you manage your physical symptoms. Chapter 6 discuss-es arthritis medications, and Chapter 7 is about managing your arthritis pain. Chapters 9 through 12 cover various aspects of exer-cise, and Chapter 13 will help you learn how to protect your joints and conserve your energy.

With good physical health-management habits in place, you will have the energy and will to address the other aspects of total wellness shown in Figure 8.1, such as emotional health, social rela-tionships, life roles, and lifestyle.

Table 8.1
Factors That Influence Health

YOU MAY NOT BE ABLE TO CONTROL	YOU CAN CONTROL
✦ Heredity	✦ Diet
✦ Environment	✦ Exercise
✦ Gender	✦ Rest
✦ Age	✦ Stress
	✦ Attitude

Emotional Health

Having a chronic, often painful condition like arthritis can have a negative effect on your emotions. If you are in pain and your usual activities are curtailed by immobility or discomfort, the results may be stress, depression, anxiety, or loss of self-esteem. Just as you have a responsibility to care for yourself physically, you need to care for yourself emotionally. It is natural, when you are first informed that you have a chronic condition, to be anxious and fearful about the future and about the effects of arthritis on your lifestyle and independence.

Taking care of your emotional health is just as important as taking care of your physical health.

Making sure that you get the emotional support that you need can be as important as anything else that you do to manage your condition. Interestingly, many of the things that you do for your emotional health have beneficial effects on your physical well-being. Physical activity or stress-management exercises such as meditation have been shown to benefit both your physical and emotional fitness. Taking positive action to deal with your emotions allows you to accept your condition and move forward with your treatment plan. Chapter 14 provides additional information about coping with the emotional impact of having arthritis, while Chapter 15 advises you on how to remain intimately close to your partner.

Social Relationships

Studies have shown that people who have good social support from family and friends cope better with their arthritis, experience less depression, and enjoy a more positive outlook. Social support has even been shown to decrease the level of pain and degree of disability a person may experience.

One of the challenges of dealing with arthritis is maintaining your pre-diagnosis social relationships and activities. Your relationships with others are naturally affected by how you react to having arthritis. If you have arthritis, you may have days when pain and fatigue seem to overtake you, and you simply want to withdraw from previously enjoyed activities with your friends. It may be that you can no longer go on hikes with friends or play some of the sports you enjoyed in the past. You may feel that because of your limitations, your value as a member of your social group is somehow diminished.

**People who have good social support from family
and friends cope better with their arthritis.**

Your reactions to pain and limited mobility will influence your relationships with friends. If you allow your symptoms to take control of your life, you may experience social isolation. This is something that you should avoid, because social support has been shown to be critically important in coping with arthritis. Your friends can be a source of help and encouragement to you as well as a distraction, bringing great pleasure into your life, but they may not understand the challenges that you face in adjusting to your arthritis. They may "kill you with kindness" or be fearful of asking you to participate in case you are not feeling well. You need to take the lead and communicate to them about what you would find helpful from them. There are proven strategies you can adopt to stay socially engaged and maintain healthy relationships with your family, friends, and coworkers. These strategies are discussed in more detail in Chapters 14 and 16.

Life Roles

Life roles are the activities that we perform. They define how we see ourselves and how others see us. They include our employment status, spousal relationship, parenting responsibilities, educational activities, and community involvement. Our sense of self-worth is strongly tied to our life roles. Sometimes we choose our life roles and prepare ourselves for them by getting an education, learning particular skills, or pursuing a career. At other times, these roles (such as that of caregiver to an elderly parent) are imposed upon us by a death in the family or a financial or health crisis.

When arthritis affects an individual's ability to fulfill one or more of his or her roles, temporarily or permanently, it can be very distressing to the individual and disruptive to family members.

Changes in life roles are challenging for everyone—not just people with arthritis.

If your role within the family changes due to your physical limitations, the roles of other family members may change in response. For example, if you previously did all the meal preparation but are now having difficulty lifting pots or peeling vegetables, another family member may need to take over those tasks. Or if you were the main wage earner in a physically demanding job, and arthritis has impaired your ability to do that job, other family members may need to take on extra financial responsibility or cut back on costs. Many families require help to adjust to changes like these. Suggestions are offered in Chapter 14 regarding ways you and your family can adjust to the shifts in roles and responsibilities that may take place.

Lifestyle

Of the many factors that contribute to your well-being, the one over which you have the most control is lifestyle. Physical activity, eating habits, weight control, stress management, and alcohol and tobacco use are things over which you have direct control. Although at times you may need help and encouragement, ultimately you have control because you can make and act upon personal choices in these areas.

**You can make the choices that
determine your lifestyle!**

Factors over which you may not have as much control include the environments in which you live and work and the stress that enters your life when unforeseen events such as illness occur (Table 8.1). If you have had a very busy and active lifestyle, having arthritis may mean that you need to slow it down, but it doesn't mean that you have to give it up! In fact, because inactivity can make the effects of arthritis worse and may lead to other health problems, it would be wise to do all you can to maintain a moderate level of activity.

It is estimated that 30 percent of people with arthritis are inactive. Don't fall into the trap of thinking that arthritis is a good excuse to be sedentary, overweight, or adopt any sort of unhealthy lifestyle. Be sure to take the time to examine your lifestyle and to adopt healthy behaviors that can help improve your overall wellness. Chapter 16 examines ways in which you can adapt your lifestyle to improve your health and wellness. Maintaining and enhancing your current health is at least as important as striving for a cure when you are ill.

HOW CAN I PREVENT DISABILITY?

The World Health Organization (WHO) describes "impairment" as loss or abnormality of an anatomical structure or function. For example, if you have arthritis in your knees, the resulting lack of movement is impairment. Impairment such as this can lead to loss of function, or disability. The term "disability" refers to problems an individual may have in carrying out daily activities or life situations. If your knee is immobile, the disability might be that you are unable to rise from a normal chair. Figure 8.2 illustrates how arthritis can lead to changes that result in disability and restrict normal activities.

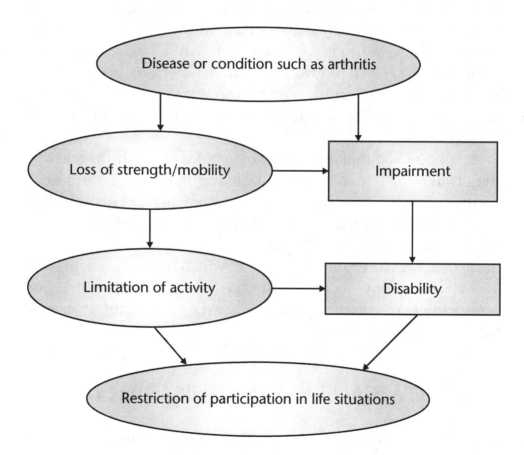

Figure 8.2
Arthritis can lead to impairment and disability and can limit your participation in life's activities. But you may be able to control whether or not this impairment leads to disability.

Whether a person with arthritis is disabled or not depends on many factors: the extent of the arthritis, whether it can be controlled by medications, the emotional impact of the condition, the way the disease affects lifestyle choices and life roles, and the availability of social or workplace support.

Who Is Disabled?

Consider two women with severe rheumatoid arthritis (RA), each taking the same medication. Both women have similar significant impairment of mobility and strength, yet they differ from each other in terms of how disabled they are by their condition.

Mrs. A. is forty-eight years old. She cares for her husband and two young daughters. Her interests are cooking, sewing, and volunteer work in a library, where she stocks the bookshelves. She lives in a two-story house with a laundry room in the basement. Her hands, knees, feet, and ankles are badly affected with RA, and she has difficulty with housecleaning and stair climbing as well as kitchen activities. Using scissors and pinning fabric are troublesome and have hampered her ability to sew. She is very anxious to resume her previous active lifestyle. In her current environment and life role, Mrs. A. would be considered very disabled by her arthritis.

Mrs. B. is sixty-seven years old and lives with her husband in a small apartment. Access to the building lobby is on the ground floor, and there is an elevator. She enjoys reading and playing bridge. She has limited movement in her knees and hips, shoulders, wrists, and fingers due to RA. She has cleaning help, and her husband and she share meal-preparation and laundry responsibilities. She has adapted her clothing and made modifications to her chairs and her bathroom. She is able to take short recreational walks in the neighborhood, using a cane and supportive shoes. She states that she has no current problems apart from episodes of joint pain. Mrs. B. would likely not be considered disabled, since her arthritis is not significantly limiting her desired level of activity.

Mrs. A's impairments are greatly disabling, given her living environment, life roles, and hobbies, while Mrs. B's impairments are not significant, since she lives in an environment that allows her to participate in a lifestyle that is satisfying to her. These are two examples of how differently rheumatoid arthritis can affect individual lives and their reactions to the disease.

As we said at the beginning of the chapter, you probably have little or no control over whether or not you experience impairment. But what these two stories demonstrate is that you may be able to control whether or not this impairment leads to disability.

Taking Action to Prevent Disability

Prevention of disability when you have arthritis begins with identifying those activities that are difficult, cause increased pain, or are unsafe, and exploring different ways of doing these activities so that you minimize the risk of disability. Take the example of being unable to rise from a chair as a result of knee problems. There are a number of ways to approach this impairment. For example, by raising the height of the chair and by doing exercises to increase mobility and strength, you can reduce or eliminate the disability. By taking action, you have accomplished two things: You have controlled the environment in which you live or work, and you have taken a first step in eliminating the disability, because the exercise will help you overcome your impairment.

Devices such as canes, wrist supports, and higher seating not only make activities easier, they also reduce the stress on vulnerable joints and prevent further stress or injury. Avoiding heavy lifting, poor posture, and activities that stress the joints can also help reduce your risk of disability. There are many other simple ways to take good care of your joints. Chapter 13 contains information on how you can safeguard your joints and save your energy.

In the workplace, you may need to work with your employer to make modifications to your workspace after you are diagnosed. There may also be ways to adjust your work hours or schedule so that you can remain productive and involved in your job. Occupational therapists frequently consult in the workplace to make it possible for employees with arthritis to work safely and effectively. Legislation has been passed both in the United States and Canada that covers the obligations of employers with respect to workers who need modifications in the work environment. See the resources section for more information on whom you can contact about this topic.

Looking Forward

This chapter provided an overview of how many aspects of an individual's life can be affected by the onset of arthritis and how these aspects are interrelated. A wellness approach to life and living can make it possible to have a full and satisfying life if you make the choice to have a positive attitude, adopt a healthy lifestyle, maintain and build social and family relationships, and make changes in your health habits and your environment. In addition, it is also important to see your health care providers regularly so that they can keep track of your general health and give you information and support in making good decisions. The content in Part II, Getting Healthy and Staying Well, will introduce you to concrete strategies to increase your activity level and take care of yourself so that you can live a full and active life with arthritis.

Chapter 9

Why Should I Exercise?

Arthritis pain would seem to be a perfect excuse to avoid exercise. However, research has shown that exercise is the cornerstone of arthritis management when combined with an effective medication regime. Exercise is also a vital part of your overall treatment program. Perhaps, most importantly, it is a part of your treatment over which you alone have complete control. *You* can decide when, where, and how to include exercise in your daily routine, making it an integral element of your healthy lifestyle. This chapter discusses the ways in which exercise benefits people with arthritis. It explains the three main types of exercise (mobility and flexibility, muscle strengthening, and fitness exercise) and provides basic exercise guidelines to help you get the most out of your exercise program.

WHAT DOES RESEARCH
TELL US ABOUT EXERCISE?

Many research studies have been carried out to examine the effectiveness of different exercise methods for people with various types of arthritis. The evidence to support the value of regular exercise and physical activity is strong and growing. Recent studies indicate that people with arthritis who do not exercise are much more likely to become deconditioned, to have more pain, and to ultimately become disabled. And yet, studies also tell us that as many as 45 percent of people with arthritis are underactive.

How Can Exercise Help Me?

Regular exercise has been shown to:

✦ Reduce disability among people with arthritis.

✦ Give people a greater sense of control over their condition.

✦ Reduce pain.

✦ Improve mood and a sense of well-being.

✦ Increase muscle strength.

✦ Increase flexibility.

✦ Improve overall fitness.

✦ Reduce the risk of other chronic illnesses, such as heart disease and some forms of cancer.

Exercise can benefit you today and in the long run!

Exercise results in even more direct benefits than those in this impressive list. It improves the nutrition to the cartilage covering the ends of the bones. Joint movement during exercise allows the cartilage to absorb nutrients and remove waste products, keeping joints healthy. Weight-bearing exercises such as walking or dancing also help to prevent osteoporosis (a disease in which bones become brittle and heal slowly). Weight-bearing exercises are activities you do on your feet that work your bones and muscles against gravity.

What Do I Need To Be a Successful Exerciser?

A recent study at the University of South Carolina looked at the factors that influence exercise participation in groups of people with arthritis: exercisers and non-exercisers. The exerciser group was made up of people who did moderate exercise on three or more days per week for thirty minutes per day or strength training or vigorous activities on three or more days per week for twenty minutes per day. The non-exerciser group exercised twenty minutes one day per week or ten minutes or less two days per week.

The results of this study identified five broad categories of barriers to exercise:

✦ Pain.

✦ Symptom management.

✦ Attitudes and beliefs.

✦ Lack of support.

✦ Lack of programs.

The main barrier to exercise in both groups was pain. However, exercisers indicated that they had the knowledge and coping skills to alter their programs and continue even when they experienced pain. Non-exercisers appeared to have less knowledge and lacked the skills to modify the exercise routine when pain affected their efforts.

The results also identified the enablers and the benefits of exercise:

+ Pain relief.

+ Improved mobility.

+ Improved independence and mood.

+ Social support and advice.

+ Programs with knowledgeable instructors.

Exercisers reported more motivation in the categories of pain relief and symptom management than did the non-exercisers. Their attitudes and beliefs were more positive, and they reported improved mood and a belief that exercise helped them to maintain independence. Both groups felt that support and encouragement helped to motivate them. Specific advice on types of exercises and programs was viewed as a very important factor in encouraging participants to exercise. Similarly, both groups identified that the presence of knowledgeable instructors and opportunities to exercise with others was valuable in helping them to maintain their exercise schedule.

The findings of this study are helping health-care professionals to understand the experiences and beliefs about exercise in people with arthritis and support the development of arthritis-specific programs within communities. These findings show that while exercise has proven benefits for arthritis patients, knowledge about adaptations for pain and support from professionals and peers are crucial to compliance. If you are ready to start exercising, doing all you can to stay motivated and informed will help you stick with the program and reap the benefits.

In self-management programs, pain management and exercise have been identified as the most important and beneficial aspects of the treatment program. This suggests that if you have arthritis, it is important for you to learn about exercise and its benefits.

People with arthritis should ask their health-care providers for advice on suitable exercise programs and ask for written material and support to begin and to maintain regular exercise. The patient-led Arthritis Self-Management Program, conducted across the United States and Canada, provides education and support to people with arthritis and promotes a lifestyle that includes exercise (see the resources section).

GETTING STARTED

If your lifestyle included regular exercise or physical activity prior to your diagnosis, having arthritis is a great reason to maintain that regular exercise program. In light of your diagnosis, you may wish to get advice on ways to adapt your current program to include arthritis-specific exercises into your normal routine, or to substitute one form of recreation for another. A physical therapist or other health-care professional experienced in arthritis management can help you to tailor your exercise to your specific needs. You are already one step ahead of the game, because your lifestyle already includes regular exercise. Keep it up!

If, on the other hand, you have not exercised regularly before or you are unsure of how to start or how to exercise safely, now is the perfect time to begin. Before you start, discuss your plans to begin exercising with your health-care provider, especially if you have any other health condition, in order to determine whether you are physically ready to begin.

You should see a physical therapist before starting an exercise program if you have:

✦ Not been accustomed to regular exercise.

✦ Severe or very active arthritis.

✦ Particularly troublesome joints.

✦ Fear of exercise because of arthritis.

✦ Insufficient information on types of safe exercise and how to begin.

✦ Recently undergone joint surgery.

A physical therapist can help you to plan, set goals, assess your progress, and, most importantly, to exercise safely.

Planning Is Important

Whether you are an old hand at exercise, completely new to exercise , or somewhere in between, a good exercise program requires planning, goal setting, and progress assessment. Arthritis is usually with you for many years; therefore, when you are considering your exercise goals, it is wise to look at the long-term gains that you may make by increasing flexibility, strength, and endurance.

As you plan your exercise program, consider the barriers to exercise that may apply to you, and think of ways to overcome these barriers. Also consider the enablers that can help you to stay motivated and on track. Ask your family and friends for support and encouragement. They may want to go for walks with you, join you in an exercise class, or accompany you on a bike ride. Look within your community for arthritis exercise programs that are suitable for you. The Arthritis Foundation and the Arthritis Society can help you find appropriate programs, and many communities have warm pools and offer exercise programs in warm water specifically designed for people with arthritis. People attending these exercise groups or pool programs enjoy the support of the other participants and the instructors.

Exercising with friends is more fun!

You might also consider joining a gym or a fitness facility. Before signing on and paying what can sometimes be a large sum, do some research. Ask questions about the qualifications of the leaders, the types of programs they offer, and whether they offer trial memberships. A trial membership will give you the opportunity to find out for yourself whether this is the best environment for you. Some gyms offer discounts to certain insurance companies or to senior citizens. Check for special offers.

Setting Goals

Many people find it helpful to set exercise goals to help them stay motivated. As they reach one goal, they then set another. It can help to write out the goals, imposing a time line, and being specific so that you will know when you have reached the goal. Be smart and realistic as you set the goals. If you have not walked farther than the distance between the living room and the kitchen in the past six months, it would be unrealistic to set a goal of walking around the block tomorrow!

Start slowly. For example, you may set an initial goal of walking two blocks. If you don't experience any increased pain or swelling, the next time, try four blocks. As you progress, though, you may need to get out of your comfort zone at some point just to find out how much is too much. Gradually increase your time or distance.

Reward yourself every time you achieve a goal!

Reward yourself for goals achieved. The reward can be anything from gold stars on your exercise chart to a night out at the movies.

HOW MUCH SHOULD I EXERCISE?

Arthritis experts agree that thirty minutes of moderate exercise done three to five times a week is the key to success. The exercises should include range-of-motion, strengthening, and endurance exercises. The exercise does not need to be done all at one time, which is good news if scheduling or fatigue are factors that tend to limit your exercising schedule. Studies have shown that three ten-minute sessions a day provide results that are just as good as one thirty-minute session. The regularity and the amount of energy expended are the things that count.

If you have been unaccustomed to exercising, you may want to work up to thirty minutes gradually by starting out with five- to ten-minute sessions several times a day and increasing the time of each session as you become stronger and more mobile. Some people with arthritis report that exercising just a few minutes in the morning helps their mobility and makes it easier to start the day. If you haven't exercised regularly for a while, you may feel some muscle stiffness or tenderness in your joints, as well as some tiredness at the end of the day. However, you will notice improvement in your endurance and a decrease of soreness as you continue to be active.

If you have joints that are particularly swollen and painful, you may want to apply ice before and after you exercise. Follow the *two-hour pain rule*. If after an exercise or activity you have pain or swelling in one or more joints for longer than two hours, this may indicate that you have done the exercise too many times, too vigorously, or incorrectly, or that you need to avoid that particular exercise or activity and talk to an expert before resuming it. Don't stop exercising. Just do fewer repetitions less vigorously, or exercise for a shorter time the next day.

Start slowly, balance rest with activity, and remember the two-hour pain rule.

Steady, slow, and consistent effort will help you achieve your goals. You also need to balance exercise with rest. Give yourself breaks throughout the day. You will need time to compensate for the extra energy it takes to carry out your exercise program. Rest periods will help you to store energy for the tasks you need to do and the activities that you enjoy. This will require some planning on your part, but be sure that exercise is a priority in your life. You can read more tips for planning a fitness program in Chapter 12.

Special Considerations

If you have fibromyalgia, there may be an increase in pain after exercise that takes some time to lessen. When this happens, you should use other techniques that you have found helpful to manage the pain. Nevertheless, you need to persevere and stick to your exercise program. The pain from weak, stiff muscles makes the symptoms of fibromyalgia worsen.

For children with arthritis, exercise is critical. Many children "outgrow" their arthritis in adolescence. If they do not carry out regular stretching of tight tissues or fail to exercise their muscles, growth disturbances may occur that will leave them with deformities or restricted movements. These conditions are preventable if children follow a regular routine of exercise. Children should be encouraged to be as active as possible with few restrictions apart from taking necessary precautions in contact sports.

WHAT ARE THE THREE TYPES OF EXERCISE?

People with arthritis should, just like medal-winning athletes, put their body to work every day, doing a variety of exercise activities. This approach stimulates the body, incorporating different muscle groups, stretching tightened structures around the joints, and moving the joint surfaces across each other to improve nutrition to the joints and improve mobility. There will, of course, be a difference between you and a professional athlete in terms of intensity and duration of exercise, but just like them, you need to use it or lose it when it comes to fitness.

Exercises to Improve Mobility and Flexibility

Exercises to improve mobility and flexibility are also referred to as range-of-motion (ROM) and stretching exercises. This type of exercise helps to maintain or restore normal joint motion and to relieve the stiffness that is common in arthritis.

Each of the joints in the body has what is known as a "normal range of movement" and is moved through that range by the muscles that act on the joint. In arthritis, the pain and inflammation can result in tightness of these muscles and contractures (shortening and toughening) of the tissues surrounding the joint. If the joint is not regularly moved through its normal range, these tissues can become tighter and shorter, restricting movement. The tightness and shortening of muscle fibers are major causes of pain in arthritis. ROM exercises can help prevent that pain.

Stretching exercises help to preserve the normal flexibility in muscles and tendons. Slow stretches, held for twenty to thirty seconds, help to lengthen muscle fibers and thus relieve the pain. ROM exercises and stretching exercises together serve as the perfect "warm-up" prior to muscle-strengthening exercises and fitness activities. See Chapter 10 for more information on how to include ROM and stretching exercises in your daily schedule.

Exercises to Build and Maintain Muscle Strength

Muscles provide support and stability to a joint. Weak muscles put the joints at risk of injury or damage, because the joints cannot sustain the forces to which we subject them when we carry out our daily activities. Strong muscles protect the joints. And with strong muscles, less energy is needed to perform tasks.

**Strong muscles protect joints and
help us to save energy.**

There are two primary reasons for the loss of muscle strength in arthritis patients. The first is the natural inclination to limit the use of joints because of pain. Muscles lose their strength and their mass if they are not used. This is referred to as muscle wasting or muscle atrophy. The second reason for loss of strength is a series of events. These events begin when the pain of arthritis causes a spasm in the muscles that flex the joints (referred to as the *flexor* muscles). At the same time, the action of the muscles that extend a joint (referred to as the *extensor* muscles) is inhibited. This results in a muscle power imbalance. This may cause the flexor muscles to go into "overdrive" and tighten in a shortened position, preventing the joint from moving through its normal range of motion. At the same time, the extensor muscles, inhibited by pain signals from the nervous system, become weak and lose their ability to extend the joint.

To increase muscle strength and prevent muscle wasting, resistance exercise is required. The two types of resistance exercise commonly recommended to build muscle strength are referred to as isometric and isotonic exercises. In isometric exercises, the muscle is contracted strongly, but the joint is not moved. These exercises are safe and useful for building strength around a painful joint. Isotonic exercises incorporate resistance using weights or elastic fitness bands while a joint is moved through its range of motion. It is wise to get the guidance of a physical therapist or other experienced person before beginning an isotonic exercise program. See Chapter 11 for more detailed information on these types of exercises.

Exercises to Improve Fitness and Endurance

Exercises to improve fitness and endurance include any activities that use the large muscles of your body—the legs, the arms, and the trunk—in rhythmic, continuous motion. These exercises are proven to benefit your heart, your lungs, your blood circulation, your energy, and your mood. You often hear this type of exercise referred to as *aerobic* exercise, because it enhances circulatory and respiratory efficiency and thus increases the body's oxygen consumption. These activities increase your heart rate and the rate at which you breathe, although they should not make you dizzy or cause difficulty with breathing.

Walking, swimming, cycling, dancing, gardening, and even vacuuming are examples of fitness and endurance activities. There are countless other examples of this type of exercise, and the best thing about them is that they can be very enjoyable and can be done with your family, friends, or others with arthritis. They are also a great reason to get outside during nice weather. As you participate in fitness and endurance exercises, your mood and sense of well-being will improve. This is because these types of activities stimulate the release of "feel good" opiates in your body. See Chapter 12 for more information on this type of exercise.

GENERAL EXERCISE POINTERS

These helpful pointers can help you no matter what type of exercise you are doing. You can also read more about general fitness practices in Chapter 12.

+ Rather than taking extra pain medication prior to exercising, time your exercise so that you do it at the time of day when your medication is the most effective. Taking extra pain medication may mask an important indicator that you are doing more than you should.

+ Be sure to invest in good, supportive footwear that will protect your feet and ankles and allow you to move in comfort.

+ You do not need to purchase expensive exercise equipment in order to succeed. Complicated, elaborate exercise equipment can be costly and may be inappropriate for your needs. Talk to your physical therapist before buying any potentially unnecessary and expensive machine.

✦ Remember that your health-care providers are there to coach you and to cheer you on.

✦ Community-based exercise and recreational activities such as yoga, tai chi, Pilates, or dance classes, as well as many sporting activities, can be safe and provide social and physical benefits. Consult your health-care professional about those that either need to be adapted or could pose a risk of harm to your joints.

Excellent information on exercise in arthritis is available through the Arthritis Foundation and The Arthritis Society in the form of printed materials on their web sites. Exercise videotapes are also available from many sources. People with Arthritis Can Exercise (PACE), Levels 1 and 2, can be ordered online through the Arthritis Foundation (see the resources section).

Looking Forward

This chapter has introduced you to the importance of exercising when you have arthritis. The following chapters explain, in more detail, how to carry out the three types of exercise we have just introduced. Chapter 16, which explores lifestyle habits, provides information on other potentially beneficial exercise programs and recreational activities that people with arthritis can enjoy.

Part 2

Getting Healthy and Staying Well

Chapter 10

Keeping Joints Mobile and Flexible

Most of the time, we don't even think about our joints and how they work. As we reach for a glass of water, stand up from a chair, dress ourselves, or turn a key in a lock, we don't give our joints a thought unless they are stiff or painful. That is because typically our joints are so reliable. When they are healthy, joints move smoothly by the action of muscles that surround them and allow us to perform an incredible number of activities every hour of every day.

Chapter 2 describes the changes that may take place in or around joints and result in loss of mobility and flexibility. This chapter contains information about what you can do when joints are affected by arthritis. It explains how smooth, almost effortless motion becomes difficult due to inflammation or damage to the joint surfaces or the tissues that surround the joints, like tendons and ligaments. The following content introduces range-of-motion and stretching exercises, which have been shown to relieve pain and help arthritis patients maintain or improve mobility and flexibility. Best of all, they are free, generally easy to do, and require no special equipment!

WHAT IS RANGE OF MOTION?

Each joint has a normal range of motion (ROM), which is the natural distance and direction of the movement of that joint. When we say that a person is suffering from limited ROM, it means that he or she has at least one joint that cannot move through its normal and full range of motion. There are a number of reasons why the ROM of an arthritis patient may be limited. ROM may be impaired by acute inflammation, or the joint may be distended with synovial fluid, thus restricting movement. Pain and muscle spasm can restrict movement, too. ROM can also be limited by mechanical factors such as damage to the joint surfaces that make them rough and uneven. If the joint surfaces are severely damaged, or the supporting tissues around them have become contracted, the joint may become misaligned (deformed). Over time, limited ROM can lead to permanent inability to move the joint beyond a certain fixed position. ROM exercises maintain or restore normal joint movement and relieve stiffness.

**Over time, limited ROM can lead
to permanent disability.**

Figures 10.1 to 10.16 illustrate the normal range of motion for the major joints of the body. These images should give you an idea of what to watch for if you are concerned about your range of motion becoming limited.

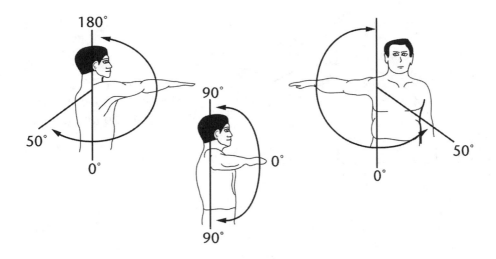

Figure 10.1
The shoulder moves forward, back, up, and down, and rotates.

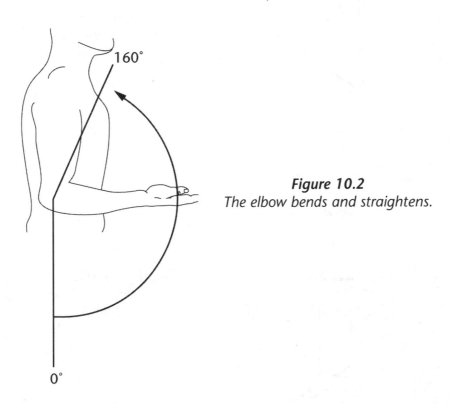

Figure 10.2
The elbow bends and straightens.

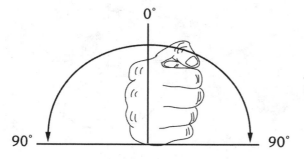

Figure 10.3
The elbow moves to turn the palm up and down.

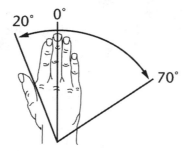

Figure 10.4
The wrist moves from side to side.

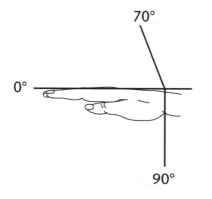

Figure 10.5
The wrist bends up and down.

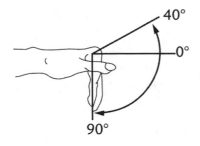

Figure 10.6
The fingers bend and straighten at the knuckles.

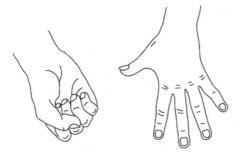

Figure 10.7
The fingers and thumb work together to grasp and manipulate objects.

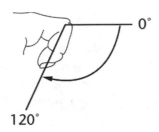

Figure 10.8
These joints allow the fingers to bend into the palm.

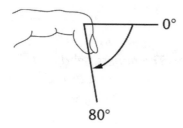

Figure 10.9
*These joints work with
the mid-joints to make
a fist.*

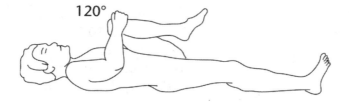

Figure 10.10
*The hip joint
flexes through
120 degrees.*

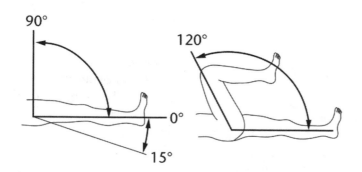

Figure 10.11
*The hip joint
bends and
straightens.*

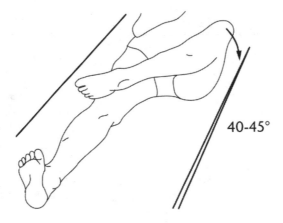

Figure 10.12
The hip joint rotates outward.

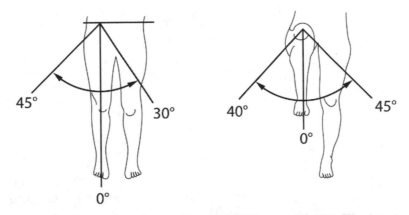

Figure 10.13
The hip joint moves the leg out to the side, inward past midline,
and rotates inward and outward.

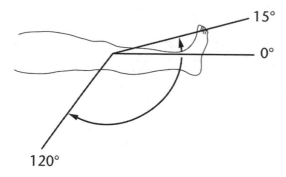

Figure 10.14
The knee bends to 120 degrees and straightens to 0 degrees and can extend beyond to 15 degrees.

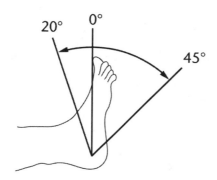

Figure 10.15
The ankle bends up and down

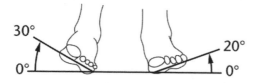

Figure 10.16
The ankle and foot move inward and outward.

WHAT ARE ROM EXERCISES?

Range-of-motion (ROM) exercises are very important; they nourish the cartilage and prevent the tightening of tissue around the joint. It may help you to understand their importance if you think of joints as hinges on a gate. If you don't open and close the gate, over time the hinges will rust shut, and if you swing on the rusting gate excessively, the hinges may wear out. If, on the other hand, you regularly open and close the gate, the hinges will neither rust nor wear out. Use it or lose it, but don't abuse it!

Joints benefit from moderate usage.

ROM exercises need to be done regularly along with stretching exercises to help you warm up before doing strengthening or fitness exercises. The number of repetitions you should do depends on whether or not the joint you plan to exercise is swollen or painful. If the joint is healthy or has arthritis but is not painful, five to ten repetitions are reasonable. If a joint is painful, do only one or two repetitions. You should do these slowly and gently, moving the joint as far as you can and holding each position at the end of the range for two to three seconds. Examples of range-of-motion exercises are illustrated in Figures 10.17-10.31. Each exercise is accompanied by a caption to assist you in understanding how to perform the action safely and effectively. The captions describe the joint(s) involved, instruct you on the starting position of the exercise, tell how the exercise is done, and inform you as to what you should watch for while doing the exercise.

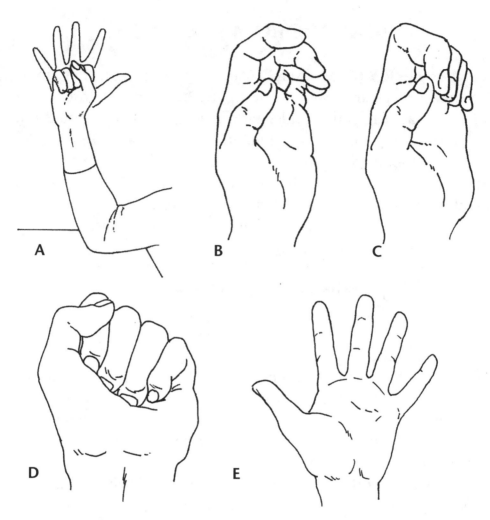

Figure 10.17
Joints Involved: Finger joints.
Starting Position: Sit with elbow supported on a table, fingers spread
wide apart, with palms of hands facing you.
How To Do the Exercise: Starting with the end joints of the fingers, and
keeping the knuckle joints straight, curl your fingertips down to touch the
crease of your palm. Fold your thumb across the fingers to make a fist.
Then straighten the fingers and thumb and stretch them apart.
Switch hands and repeat.
What To Watch For: Make sure that you curl the end joints first,
the middle joints next, then roll the tips of the fingers into the palm.

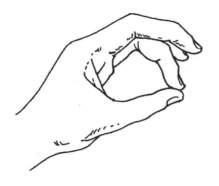

Figure 10.18
Joints Involved: *Thumb joints.*
Starting Position: *Sit with elbow at 90 degrees.*
How To Do the Exercise: *Touch the tip of your thumb to the tip of each finger in sequence, forming an "O" each time. Stretch your thumb and fingers out after each touch. Switch hands and repeat.*
What To Watch For: *Do not push with the tip of your thumb on the side of any of your fingers; just touch tip to tip.*

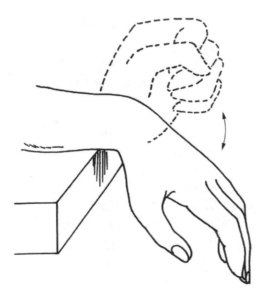

Figure 10.19
Joints Involved: *Wrist joints.*
Starting Position: *Sit with forearm supported on a table, hand relaxed, over the edge of the table.*
How To Do the Exercise: *Make a fist as you extend the wrist, relax, and let the hand drop as you extend and spread the fingers. Switch hands and repeat.*
What To Watch For: *Keep your fingers bent tightly as you extend the wrist, stretch your fingers as you drop your hand.*

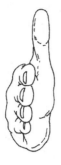
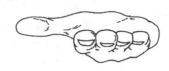
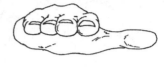

Figure 10.20
Joints Involved: Elbow joints.
*Starting Position: Sit with elbows tucked in at your sides,
fingers straight, thumbs pointing upward.*
*How To Do the Exercise: turn thumb to the outside as far as possible so
that your palm is facing upward. Then roll your hand palm down so that
your thumb is pointing inward. Imagine tracing a semicircle with your
thumbs. Switch sides and repeat.*
*What To Watch For: Keep your elbows tucked in and try to make both the
palm and the back of your hand parallel to the floor as you rotate.*

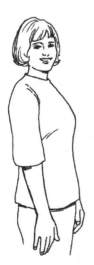
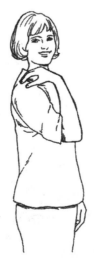

Figure 10.21
Joints Involved: Elbow joints.
*Starting Position: Stand with
your arms straight down
at your sides.*
*How To Do the Exercise: Bend
elbows and bring your hands up
to touch your shoulders. Slowly
lower your forearms to your side.
Switch sides and repeat.*
*What To Watch For: Keep your
elbows tucked close to your sides.*

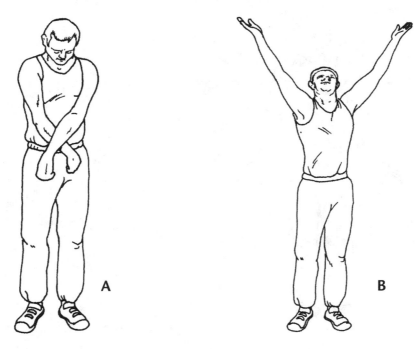

Figure 10.22
Joints Involved: Shoulder joints.
Starting Position: *Stand with your arms crossed in front at hip level, with closed fists and bent wrists.*
How To Do the Exercise: *Open your hands wide, extend the wrists, and uncross arms as you lift them up and away, leading with the thumb. Make a fist, bend your wrists, and return arms to starting position*
What To Watch For: *This exercise can also be done sitting in a straight-backed chair or lying on your back.*

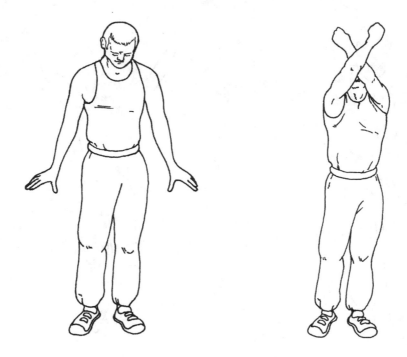

Figure 10.23
Joints Involved: Shoulder joints.
Starting Position: Stand with hands by sides away from the hips with hands wide open and facing down.
How To Do the Exercise: Make a fist, bend your wrists, and bring arms up and forward, crossing your arms at the end of movement. Open hands wide, extend your wrists, and uncross your hands as you bring them back to the starting position.
What To Watch For: Proceed as in previous exercise. Keep your fingers and wrists bent tightly as you raise your arms. Open your hands and extend your wrists as you lower your arms to your sides.

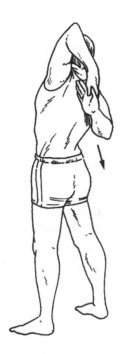

Figure 10.24
Joints Involved: *Shoulder joints.*
Starting Position: *Sit or stand.*
How To Do the Exercise: *Put your right
hand behind your back, reaching up
as far as possible. Put your left hand
behind your neck and reach down as far
as possible. Repeat putting your right
hand behind yoru neck and your
left hand behind your neck.*
What To Watch For: *Try to touch
the fingers of both hands
as you do this exercise.*

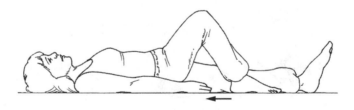

Figure 10.25
Joints Involved: *Knee joints.*
Starting Position: *Lie on your back with the knees stright.*
How To Do the Exercise: *Slide right heel toward the right butock
as far as possible, keeping the left leg straight.
Then slide the heel back down to straighten the hip and knee.
Repeat with the left leg.*
What To Watch For: *When straightening the knee, try to touch the bed or
mat with the back of your knee and then lift the heel slightly.*

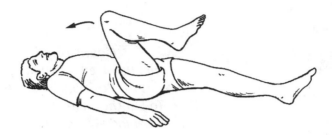

Figure 10.26
Joints Involved: *Hip joints.*
Starting Position: *Lie on your back with the knees straight.*
How To Do the Exercise: *Bend right knee up as far as possible, keeping the left leg straight, then straighten the hip and knee back to the starting position. Repeat with the left leg.*
What To Watch For: *Keep the flat of your back in touch with the bed, and try not to lift the opposite leg as you bend your hip.*

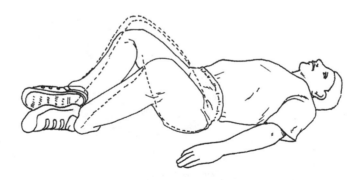

Figure 10.27
Joints Involved: *Hip joints.*
Starting Position: *Lie on your back with the knees bent and feet apart, in line with the hips.*
How To Do the Exercise: *Turn the soles of your feet to face each other and allow the knees to fall out to the side.*
What To Watch For: *Feel the stretch in your groin. Keep your back flat during the exercise.*

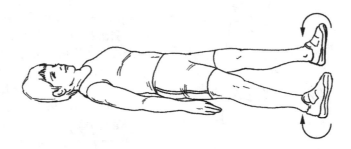

Figure 10.28
Joints Involved: *Hip joints.*
Starting Position: *Lie on your back with legs out straight and feet apart.*
How To Do the Exercise: *Roll your feet toward each other as far as possible and then away from each other as far as possible..*
What To Watch For: *Keep your back flat and your knees straight during the exercise.*

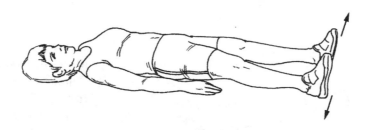

Figure 10.29
Joints Involved: *Hip joints.*
Starting Position: *Lie on your back with legs out straight, toes pointing upward.*
How To Do the Exercise: *Slide one leg out as far as possible then back to midline. Repeat with the other leg.*
What To Watch For: *Keep your toes pointing straight up.*

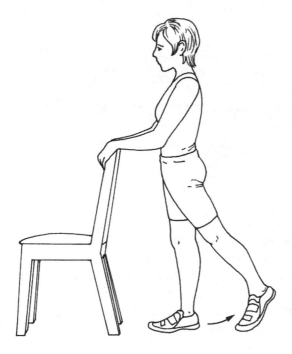

Figure 10.30
Joints Involved: *Hip joints.*
Starting Position: *Stand,. holding the edge of a table or the back of a chair at about waist height.*
How To Do the Exercise: *Keeping your knee straight, swing your right leg back as far as possible. Return to the midline and repeat to the left.*
What To Watch For: *Keep your spine straight; do not bend forward from the waist.*

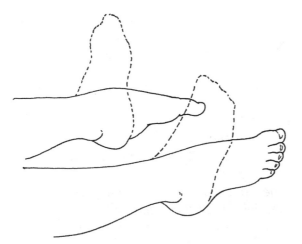

Figure 10.31
Joints Involved: *Ankle joints.*
Starting Position: *Lie down.*
How To Do the Exercise: *Point your feet downward, then upward as far as possible.*
What To Watch For: *If your knees are straight, you should feel a stretch in your calf as your feet point upward.*

WHAT ARE STRETCHING EXERCISES?

Stretching exercises are directed toward maintaining or restoring normal flexibility to the surrounding muscles and tendons of the joint. You need to do these exercises along with the ROM exercises, because, in order to be effective, the joints need the supporting tissues such as tendons, ligaments, and muscles to be flexible. Joint surfaces do not have nerve endings in them, but nerves are present in abundance in muscles, ligaments, and tendons. If these joint tissues become tight and contracted, the nerves in them can cause pain when you attempt to move a joint. Stretching exercises are similar to the range-of-motion exercises, but stretching targets the soft tissues around a joint.

Stretching exercises also should be done more slowly than ROM exercises and held for a longer time at the end of the range. Two to three repetitions of each exercise, holding for twenty to thirty seconds, are recommended if the joint is not swollen and painful. Do not bounce in your stretches. If the joint is swollen and painful, avoid the stretching exercise until the inflammation subsides. These exercises also help to improve posture and reduce the risk of injuries during other activities.

Exercise is the key to freedom of movement.

Examples of stretching exercises are illustrated in Figures 10.32 to 10.38. Each exercise is accompanied by a caption to assist you in understanding how to perform the action safely and effectively. The legend describes the joint (s) and muscle(s) involved, instructs you on the starting position of the exercise, tells how the exercise is done, and informs you about what you should watch for while doing the exercise.

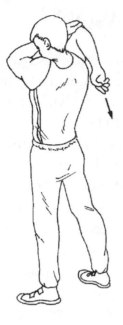

Figure 10.32
Joints and/or Muscles Involved:
Shoulder.
Starting Position:
Stand.
How To Do the Exercise: *Reach up and
over your shoulder with one arm. With the
opposite hand, push gently with the
opposite hand at the point of the elbow.
Hold the position for twenty to thirty
seconds. Repeat two to three times.*
What To Watch For:
*You should feel a pull in the muscles across
the front of the shoulder joint.*

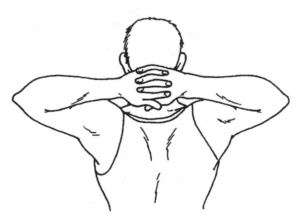

Figure 10.33
Joints and/or Muscles Involved: *Shoulder.*
Starting Position: *Stand.*
How To Do the Exercise: *Clasp your hands behind your neck. Bring your
elbows out to the side and push your shoulder blades back together. Hold
the position for twenty to thirty seconds. Repeat two to three times.*
What To Watch For: *Keep your neck straight and your elbows level with
your shoulder joints.*

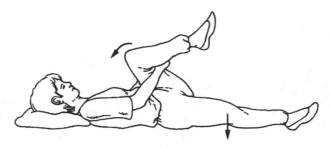

Figure 10.34
Joints and/or Muscles Involved: *Hip and lower back.*
Starting Position: *Lie with both legs straight.*
How To Do the Exercise: *Bend one knee and clasp your hands under the knee. Pull the knee up as far as possible toward the chest. Hold the position for twenty to thirty seconds. Repeat two to three times. Switch knees and repeat.*
What To Watch For: *Push your other leg down toward the floor.*

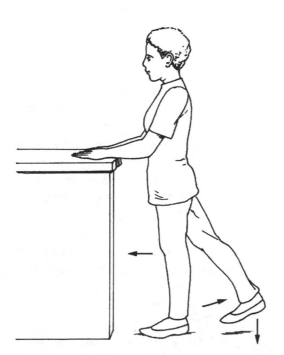

Figure 10.35
Joints and/or Muscles Involved: *Hip and calf muscles.*
Starting Position: *Stand, supported by a chair or table at approximately waist height.*
How To Do the Exercise: *Bring leg backward, keeping your knee straight. At the end of the movement, push your heel down toward the floor while bending the opposite knee. Hold the position for twenty to thirty seconds. Repeat two to three times. Switch legs and repeat.*

What To Watch For: *Keep your head up and your spine straight as the opposite knee bends. Do not lean forward.*

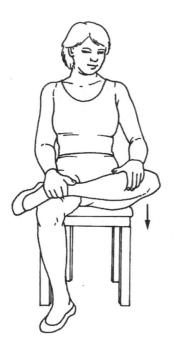

Figure 10.36
Joints and/or Muscles Involved: Hip.
Starting Position: Sit on a chair.
How To Do the Exercise: Place one ankle on top of the opposite knee. Using the hand on the same side, push down on the knee, toward the floor. Hold the position for twenty to thirty seconds. Repeat two to three times. Switch legs and repeat.
What To Watch For: Keep your weight evenly distributed on both buttocks. Feel the stretch on the inside of your thigh.

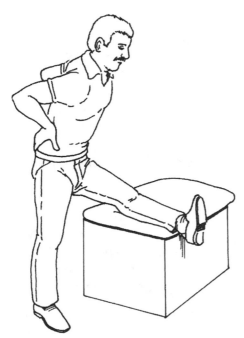

Figure 10.37
Joints and/or Muscles Involved: Knee and calf muscles.
Starting Position: Stand with one leg supported on a bench or low chair seat, heel over the edge. The chair should not be above knee height.
How To Do the Exercise: Push forward with the opposite hip and keep your back straight as you bend forward. Point your toes upward toward your body. Hold the position for twenty to thirty seconds. Repeat two to three times.
What To Watch For: Keep your knee straight. Feel the stretch behind your knee and in your calf muscles.

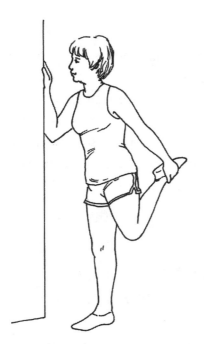

Figure 10.38
Joints and/or Muscles Involved: *Hip and muscles at the front of the thigh.*
Starting Position: *Lean against a wall with one hand, or hold onto a chair.*
How To Do the Exercise: *Grasp the top of one foot and pull it gently toward your buttock. Hold the position for twenty to thirty seconds. Repeat two to three times. Switch legs and repeat.*
What To Watch For: *Keep your spine and hips straight. Feel the stretch across the front of your hip joint and through the muscles at the front of your thigh.*

WHEN SHOULD I DO MY ROM AND STRETCHING EXERCISES?

ROM and stretching exercises need to be done daily to provide maximum benefit. You may need to do some experimenting to find out what time of day suits you best. Some people feel that if they do these exercises immediately upon getting out of bed in the morning, it helps to relieve morning stiffness. They feel that the exercises are a good way to start the day, and so they build in a little extra time for exercise in the morning. You can do exercises for your neck, shoulders, elbows, wrists, and hands while standing in a warm shower. If lack of time or fatigue is troublesome, try breaking up your exercise routine into shorter periods throughout the day.

Special Considerations

People with ankylosing spondylitis report that their symptoms are worse after rest and improve with exercise. Because of this, most patients with AS prefer to do these exercises in the morning.

Many people with osteoarthritis say that, after sitting for a period of time, it is difficult to stand up and start walking. You may find it easier if, while still sitting, you bend and stretch your knees a few times before putting your weight on them. This is like a mini warm-up.

WHERE SHOULD I DO MY ROM AND STRETCHING EXERCISES?

The best place to do these exercises is wherever you feel the most comfortable. Some people prefer to exercise in the privacy of their own home. This is convenient if you prefer to do these exercises as you begin the day or right before bed. Nearly all ROM and stretching exercises can be done lying on the bed. Some, especially the upper-body exercises, can be done while sitting. You can do hand and wrist exercises while sitting at your desk at work or watching TV.

Exercising in a group, especially in a warm pool, can allow for social interaction and encouragement. However, people often find it difficult, when they have significant morning stiffness, to get to a class or pool program early in the day. If you have a lot of fatigue, you may wish to avoid exercise programs in the evening. When you are planning your exercise sessions, try to choose programs that are held at a time of day when you feel the best.

Balance rest with exercise.

Of course, you must be aware of any potential changes in your arthritis symptoms, such as increased joint pain and stiffness or increased fatigue. If your symptoms worsen in response to exercise (remember the two-hour rule from Chapter 7?), adjust your exercise program accordingly, and remember that you need to balance exercise with rest.

HOW DO I GET STARTED WITH ROM AND STRETCHING EXERCISES?

Getting started on a regular exercise routine can be challenging, particularly if you have never been physically active before. The exercises shown in this chapter are of a general nature and are great for beginners. Your health-care team is also an excellent resource to help you figure out how to begin. Physical therapists and occupational therapists can assess your disease activity and your range of motion. They can then help you to select exercises that are safe and tailored to your individual needs and teach you how to identify actively inflamed joints or joints with special problems. They can also teach you how to monitor your response to the exercise program and make modifications if necessary.

You can order exercise pamphlets, brochures, and videos through the Arthritis Foundation and The Arthritis Society (see the resources section), but it is still a good idea to get professional advice and assistance in learning to do these exercises. Practice makes perfect, and after a short period of instruction, you should be able to carry out these exercises unsupervised.

Plan your exercise periods so that they don't get neglected. Make a contract with yourself that includes detailed commitments for how often and how long you will exercise. Keep an exercise chart or log so that you can check your progress. After a while, you won't need this, as exercise will become just as much a part of your daily routine as brushing your teeth or taking your medication. Building exercise into your life is an excellent way for you to take control of your arthritis. Don't pass up the chance to take charge and make a very real difference in your life.

Looking Forward

ROM and stretching exercises are crucial in the battle to keep your joints mobile and flexible. Along with the two other types of exercise that we discuss in Chapters 11 and 12, they will help you attain wellness. The following two chapters offer you guidance on building your muscle strength to support your joints and incorporating aerobic-fitness activities that can improve your cardiovascular health and endurance as well as your sense of well-being.

Chapter 11

Building and Maintaining Your Muscle Strength

The human body contains three different types of muscles; each type has a different function. Cardiac muscles are located in the heart and produce the pumping action for which this organ is known; their action is *involuntary (you have no control over this action)*. Smooth muscles are mostly found in visceral organs (like your stomach and intestines); their action is also *involuntary*. Skeletal or striated muscles help move all synovial joints; their action is *voluntary (you have control over this action)*. Chapter 11 explains the action and function of skeletal muscles, how they change due to arthritis, and how to maintain and increase their strength. Chapter 12 will show you how to build up endurance in your muscles.

SKELETAL MUSCLE ACTION
AND FUNCTION

Skeletal muscles are voluntary—they contract and relax when you want them to. There are two types of contractions, isotonic and isometric. During isotonic contraction, a muscle changes in length as it contracts. The muscle can contract as it lengthens, as when you lower a weight held in your hand, or it can contract as it shortens, as when you lift that weight in your hand. During isometric contraction, a muscle maintains its length as it contracts. Isotonic muscle contraction results in joint movement, whether it is lengthening (eccentric contraction) or shortening (concentric contraction), while isometric muscle contraction helps to stabilize your joints or body parts.

A muscle or groups of muscles can move joints in one plane, as when you straighten a finger; in two planes, as when you bring food to your mouth; or in three planes, as when you serve a tennis ball. Certain movements require the muscles to work very hard—for example, when you lift a heavy weight. Other movements put minimal demand on the muscles, such as swinging your arms as you walk. For a muscle to work hard, it has to be strong. In order to do things like swing your arms as you walk, muscles also need endurance.

Range-of-Muscle Contraction

The range of a muscle's contraction varies depending on its size and location. For example, the hamstring muscles are among the longest in the body, and due to their location at the back of the thigh, they both bend the knee and extend the hip, thus acting on two joints. When the hamstrings contract to bend the knee and extend the hip fully, they are at their shortest contraction or range. When the knee is extended and the hip is bent, the hamstrings are at their longest stretch or range.

A muscle that is fully contracted or fully stretched does not work efficiently and will lose the strength of its contraction. If strong resistance is applied to a fully stretched muscle, its fibers can be put at risk of tearing. To prevent this, the muscle tends to relax reflexively. If strong resistance is applied when a muscle is fully contracted or is at its shortest, it is at a mechanical disadvantage due to its acute angle of pull and may cause a cramp.

**Muscles are strongest when they
contract in their middle range.**

A muscle is at its strongest when it is working in its middle range, where the muscle work is risk-free. The resisted muscle-strengthening exercises described in this chapter will mostly be halfway between full contraction and full stretch—in other words, in the middle range where your muscles are at their strongest.

Muscles Work in Groups

Muscles work cooperatively so that the action they produce is smooth and well coordinated. Let's consider the knee for a moment. If you straighten your knee, that action is produced by the contraction of the quadriceps muscles at the front of the thigh. Because the quadriceps is the prime mover for that action, that muscle is called the **agonist**. The hamstring muscles at the back of the thigh must relax to permit the quadriceps to extend the knee. The relaxing hamstrings are referred to as the **antagonists**. When the hamstrings in the return movement bend the knee, they become the agonists, and the relaxing quadriceps becomes the antagonist. If both muscles contract at the same time, there will be no movement. Therefore, in order for the quadriceps to extend the knee, the hamstrings have to relax, and for the hamstrings to bend the knee, the quadriceps have to relax. In patients with inflammatory or painful arthritis, the agonists such as the quadriceps have to overcome the protective muscle spasm of the hamstrings that may become tight while trying to hold the knee in a bent position to prevent painful movements.

Another group of muscles cooperates with the agonists during a movement; again to make their action smooth and coordinated, these are called the **synergists**, which work isotonically. A fourth group of muscles works with the agonists to help stabilize a related joint and prevent it from flopping around. These are called **fixators**, and they work isometrically. When you bend your elbow against resistance, you will be aware of contractions in your shoulder muscles. These are the synergists that are working isotonically to assist the action of the agonists, as well as the fixators that are stabilizing the shoulder girdle by working isometrically. Together they add strength and coordination to the action of the agonists.

Muscles work in groups to produce powerful, smooth, and coordinated movements.

You can see what a complex series of events is involved in muscle movement. In order to help your body move well, muscle-strengthening exercises must target not only the agonists, but also the synergists or fixators that contribute to any given action. At the same time, the antagonists have to be trained to relax when the agonists are working.

How Does the Inflammatory Process of Arthritis Weaken Skeletal Muscles?

The main objective of skeletal-muscle strengthening exercises is to restore or maintain the best possible level of strength in those muscles that support and act on joints affected by arthritis. These muscles can become weak for a variety of interconnected reasons.

The soft tissues around a joint are rich with sensory nerve endings that transmit pain sensations to the brain or central nervous system. When a joint is inflamed, it fills with synovial fluid that stretches the soft tissues enclosing a joint, much like a balloon pumped with air stretches its rubbery walls. The sensory nerve endings register this stretch and alert your brain that something is not right. These signals are interpreted by the brain as pain sensations, warning your body to protect these soft tissues from over-stretching and becoming injured.

If you move an inflamed joint, the extra fluid is dispersed throughout the joint. In certain positions, such as a slightly bent knee, joints can accommodate more fluid and therefore put less stress on the soft tissues. On the other hand, if you straighten that knee or fully bend it, it accommodates less fluid and tends to compress the extra fluid within the joint, exerting more pressure on the soft tissues and causing more pain. This is the reason why arthritis patients tend to hold an inflamed or swollen joint in certain positions—they are trying to avoid pain by doing so. The amount of movement in a swollen joint depends on the amount of extra fluid; the range of movement is lessened and the pain is greater the more fluid there is in a joint. If movement is painful, people stop moving, and the muscles acting on painful joints are not used frequently. Since muscles need to work hard to remain strong, weaker contractions or diminished loads result in disuse and subsequently muscle atrophy or weakness.

**The pain of joint inflammation can put
a stop to the work of the muscles.**

To add insult to injury, when the brain perceives pain coming from a diseased or injured joint, it sends messages to the muscles acting on this joint to lessen their voluntary action and ability to contract. This process is known as *reflex inhibition*. This reflex can be so strong as to obliterate, temporarily, the ability of the affected muscle to voluntarily contract. To counter the forces acting to weaken your muscles, it is important that you engage in strengthening exercises to restore or maintain the best possible level of strength in those muscles that support and act on joints affected by arthritis.

WHAT DO I NEED TO KNOW BEFORE I BEGIN MY MUSCLE-STRENGTHENING PROGRAM?

Before you plan an exercise program to increase or maintain muscle strength, consider the following points:

✦ If the joints targeted for exercise are inflamed, make every effort to control the inflammation using appropriate, prescribed anti-inflammatory medications taken orally or injected into the joint.

✦ Schedule a few sessions with a physical therapist before starting your exercise program to help you select the appropriate type of exercise that will meet your needs.

✦ You do not want the condition of the joint to be worsened by the exercise.

✦ Joint swelling and pain that continue for two hours after exercise are indications of excessive use, especially if these symptoms increase during the subsequent twenty-four-hour period.

✦ Do not exercise the muscles to fatigue.

✦ A warm-up program of range-of-motion exercises and stretches must precede strengthening exercises. See Chapter 10 for more information on these types of exercise.

✦ The starting position for a particular exercise depends on the location of the muscles and joints exercised, on your ability to maintain a certain position, and on the severity of the arthritis. Exercises can be done in lying, sitting, or standing positions.

✦ To increase strength, a muscle must work against a load or resistance. Resistance can be provided by your own body, a firm object, another person, a heavy object (as when you lift weights), or by elastic objects such as springs or elastic rubber strips.

✦ The amount of resistance you should use depends on the condition of the joint. Muscles acting on acutely inflamed joints require minimal resistance when they are exercised isometrically and no resistance when exercised isotonically. Also, they require only one to two repetitions to keep the joint mobile. On non-acutely inflamed joints, aim for maximal isometric contractions and submaximal contractions (anything less than the greatest contraction possible) that require an 80 percent effort for isotonic work.

✦ The number of repetitions for isotonic exercise can be five to ten repetitions to start, progressing to a maximum of fifteen repetitions; for isometric exercise, three to four repetitions are advised.

IS ISOMETRIC OR ISOTONIC EXERCISE BETTER FOR MY ARTHRITIS?

The choice between isometric and isotonic exercise depends on the purpose of the exercise and on whether the joint is inflamed.

The Benefits of Isometric Exercises

Isometric exercise at submaximal effort (less than your greatest effort) offers greater protection to an acutely inflamed or unstable joint. Isometric exercise can benefit most people. When no joint inflammation is present, three or four repetitions of isometric muscle contractions at maximal effort (the greatest effort you are capable of), each held for six seconds, can achieve a remarkable increase in muscle strength of about 30 percent in just over a two-week period. The amount of resistance you work with should not exceed your ability to hold the position.

Because isometric training also helps in the performance of isotonic movements, it can be a useful substitute for isotonic muscle work while the joint is inflamed. A word of caution about isometric exercise: Patients with heart failure or other forms of heart disease should *not* do isometric exercise, as it puts too much strain on the heart.

**Patients with heart disease
should avoid isometric exercise.**

The Benefits of Isotonic Exercises

When no joint inflammation is present, resisted isotonic muscle work at submaximal effort can also improve muscle strength significantly. It is used to train muscles for tasks that require a combination of movement and strength, such as lifting heavy objects off of the ground (concentric action), or lowering heavy objects to the ground (eccentric action). However, resisted isotonic contractions should be tailored to an individual's needs, taking into consideration factors related to age, severity of the arthritis, other medical problems, the amount of joint damage, general strength, and functional needs of the individual.

Once you have established a program, one session a day of isotonic exercise is recommended. Increase the number of repetitions and resistance to tolerance as you gain strength. Do not apply resistance across two joints; it is preferable to apply resistance to muscles acting on one joint at a time. For example, when you are applying resistance to muscles that bend the hip joint, the point of resistance should be above the knee joint and not at the ankle, which would subject the knee to undesirable force.

GETTING STARTED WITH A MUSCLE-STRENGTHENING PROGRAM

The next two sections in this chapter describe a series of isometric and isotonic exercises, starting with exercises in the lying position and progressing to upright positions. Each exercise is accompanied by a caption to assist you in understanding how to perform the action safely and effectively. The caption describes the muscles or group of muscles involved, indicates whether the exercise is isometric or isotonic, instructs you on the starting position of the exercise, tells you how the exercise is done, and informs you as to what you should watch for while doing the exercise.

These exercises must be preceded by ROM and stretching exercises as described in Chapter 10. All of the exercises are simple to perform and can be done in the comfort of your home. You may choose to do them in one setting, or split them into two or three settings on a given day. The only piece of equipment you need to purchase is an exercise band. The company Thera-band makes exercise bands that are color coded. Each color offers a different resistance to stretch. Thera-band products can be purchased from your local medical home-equipment suppliers and from some pharmaceutical chains. They can also be ordered through the Internet.

Isometric and Isotonic Strengthening Exercises

Figures 11.1 to 11.14 show a series of isometric and isotonic strengthening exercises that are recommended for people with arthritis. Most of these exercises require no outside resistance and are called isometric setting exercises. For others, the muscle contraction is resisted by pressing on an object such as a bed, table, or wall. Each isometric exercise must be repeated three or four times slowly. Be sure that you reach a maximal contraction and hold it for six seconds. Apply submaximal effort (any effort less than your greatest effort) if you are in pain or when the joint is inflamed, and maximal effort if you are not experiencing joint pain or inflammation. To avoid holding your breath while doing the exercise, breathe out gently while exerting the effort. The exercise you choose depends on the type of problem you have and what you expect to achieve by doing it.

Interspersed with isometric exercises, you will find a series of isotonic strengthening exercises that are recommended for people with arthritis. All of these exercises are self-resisted for simplicity and ease of use in your home. Do not perform resisted isotonic muscle work when joint inflammation is present. Remember to keep your movement slow and smooth; jerky movements can cause muscle strain. Breathe out gently while you are making the effort. Each exercise must be repeated five to ten times; you can increase them to a maximum of fifteen repetitions. The resistance offered to each movement should be submaximal and increased gradually.

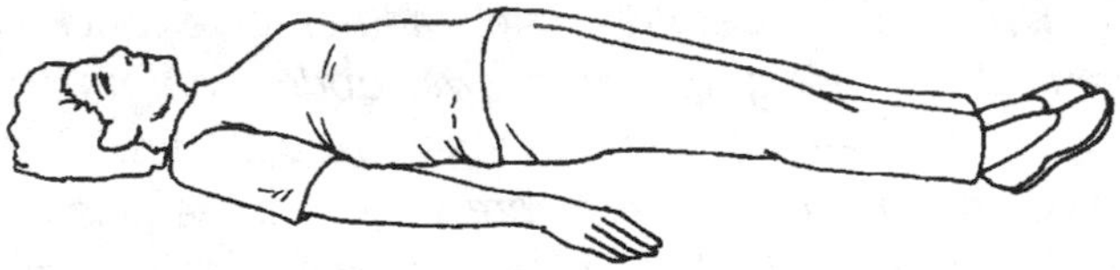

Figure 11.1
Muscle Groups Involved: *Extensors of the hips,*
back, and shoulders. Isometric work.
Starting Position: *Lie flat on back, legs apart*
and feet pointing down, arms by sides.
How To Do the Exercise: *Push heels and arms into the mat*
and tighten buttock muscles without lifting hips.
Then release tension. Repeat three or four times.
What To Watch For: *Tighten your muscles gradually.*
When you reach your maximal contraction,
hold that position for a count of six.
Breathe out slowly as you tighten muscles.

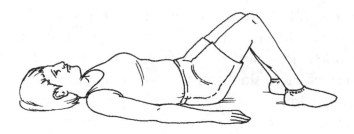

Figure 11.2
Muscle Groups Involved: *Lower abdominal muscles. Isometric work.*
Starting Position: *Lie on back with knees bent at a 90-degree angle,*
feet resting on the floor, arms by sides.
How To Do the Exercise: *Press the small of lower back against*
the mat as you tighten your lower abdominal muscles.
Then release. Repeat three or four times.
What To Watch For: *Proceed as in previous exercise (see information*
regarding Figure 11.1). The first time you do the exercise,
place your hand under the small of your lower back as you
tighten your muscles to feel how the exercise should be done.

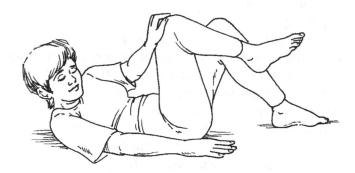

Figure 11.3
Muscle Groups Involved: *Upper and lower abdominal muscles*
and pusher muscles of your arm. Isometric work.
Starting Position: *Proceed as in previous exercise (see Figure 11.2).*
How To Do the Exercise: *Bending right hip, raise head and press with left*
outstretched hand against your bent knee. Then release. Switch sides (right
hand pressing on left knee). Repeat three or four times on each side.
What To Watch For: *Proceed as in previous exercises (see information*
regarding Figure 11.1). Discontinue exercise if it causes pain
in the lower back.

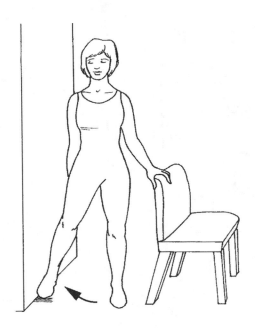

Figure 11.4
Muscle Groups Involved: *Muscles
that maintain pelvic balance
during walking. Isometric work.*
Starting Position: *Stand close to a
wall. Begin with right side facing the
wall and a foot away, and left hand
holding the back of a chair.*
How To Do the Exercise: *Move right
leg sideways, pressing the side of
right foot against the wall. Then
release. Switch sides. Repeat three
or four times on each side.*
What To Watch For: *Proceed as in
previous exercises (see information
for Figure 11.1). Keep your upper
body straight as you do the exercise.*

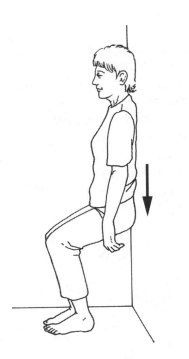

Figure 11.5
Muscle Groups Involved:
*Calf muscles, knee and hip extensors.
Isotonic work.*
Starting Position: *Stand with
back leaning against a wall,
feet slightly apart.*
How To Do the Exercise: *With back
firmly against the wall, slide down
slowly until hips and knees are at a
90-degree angle. Then straighten up
slowly. Repeat five to ten times,
progresssing to fifteen repetitions.*
What To Watch For: *You should
descend slowly as you breathe out.
Do not reach the 90-degree angle at
first if you find the exercise difficult,
but gradually progress to reach
that angle.*

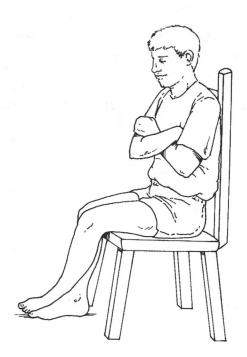

Figure 11.6
Muscle Groups Involved:
Knee extensor and knee flexor muscles. Isometric work.
Very important for walking and using stairs.
Starting Position: *Sit on a straight-backed chair, arms folded, feet resting on the floor and crossed at the ankles.*
How To Do the Exercise: *Press top leg against the bottom leg without allowing movement. Release. Switch legs and repeat sequence. Repeat three or four times on each side.*
What To Watch For: *Tighten your muscles gradually. When you reach your maximal contraction, hold that position for a count of six. Breathe out slowly as you tighten your muscles.*

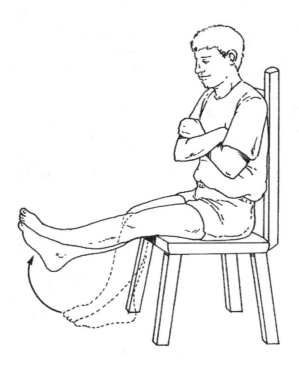

Figure 11.7
Muscle Groups Involved: *Knee extensor and knee flexor muscles. Isotonic work. Very important for walking and using stairs.*
Starting Position: *Proceed as in previous exercise (see Figure 11.6).*
How To Do the Exercise: *Resist the movement of the lower leg with the upper leg as the lower leg. Then resist the movement of the lower leg with the upper leg as it bends, bringing the legs back to the starting position. Repeat the same sequence five to ten times, progressing to fifteen repetitions.*
What To Watch For: *This isotonic exercise provides shortening muscle work for one leg (isotonic concentric) and lengthening muscle work for the other (isotonic eccentric). This is a very useful exercise. Take time to learn to do it properly.*

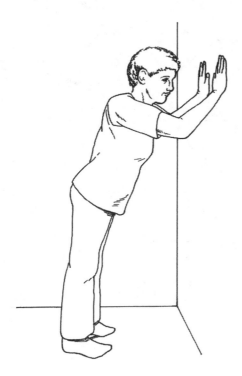

Figure 11.8

Muscle Groups Involved: Elbow and hip extensors, and muscles that control the shoulder girdle. Isotonic work.

Starting Position: Stand two feet away from a wall, and place your hands against the wall with elbows straight.

How To Do the Exercise: Lean forward as you bend your elbows, then push with your arms away from the wall, returning to starting position. Repeat five to ten times, progressing to fifteen repetitions.

What To Watch For: If your hands are severely affected with arthritis, do not do this exercise.

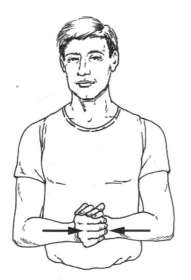

Figure 11.9

Muscle Groups Involved: Muscles that bend the wrists, elbows, and shoulders (the pectorals). Isometric work.

Starting Position: Stand or sit, upper arms by sides, elbows at right angles, palms touching.

How To Do the Exercise: Push the palm of one hand against the palm of the other hand, without allowing movement. Then release. Repeat three or four times.

What To Watch For: Tighten your muscles gradually. When you reach your maximal contraction, hold that position for a count of six. Breathe out slowly as you tighten muscles.

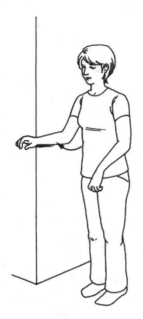

Figure 11.10
Muscle Groups Involved: *Muscles that raise and rotate the arm outward and stabilize the shoulder girdle. Isometric work.*
Starting Position: *Stand with side facing a wall, upper arms at sides, elbows bent at 90 degrees.*
How To Do the Exercise: *Press forearm against the wall, then let go. Repeat three or four times on each side.*
What To Watch For: *Proceed as in previous exercise (see information regarding Figure 11.9).*

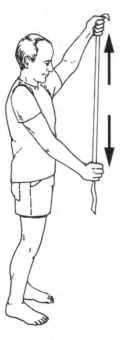

Figure 11.11
Muscle Groups Involved: *Muscles that raise the arm on one side and lower the arm on the other. Isotonic work.*
Starting Position: *Stand or sit on a firm chair, and hold the ends of an 18-inch exercise band, arms straight in front of you.*
How To Do the Exercise: *Stretch the exercise band by raising one arm with thumb pointing to the ceiling, and lowering the other with thumb pointing to the floor simultaneously. Return slowly to starting position. Repeat five to ten times, progressing to fifteen repetitions. Switch arm positions and repeat.*
What To Watch For: *If you are using colored Thera-bands, start with tan Thera-band, and as you get stronger, progress to yellow, red, and green bands, in that order.*

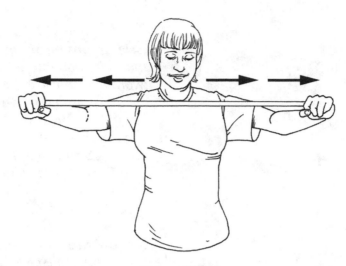

Figure 11.12
Muscle Groups Involved: *Muscles that extend and retract the shoulder.*
Starting Position: *Stand, arms raised straight out in front of you at shoulder level, elbows straight, holding the ends of an eighteen-inch exercise band.*
How To Do the Exercise: *Stretch the exercise band by moving arms horizontally and away from each other. Then return slowly to starting position. Repeat five to ten times, progressing to fifteen repetitions.*
What To Watch For: *Proceed as in previous exercise (see information regarding Figure 11.11).*

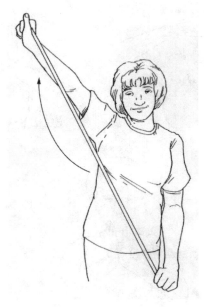

Figure 11.13
Muscle Groups Involved: *Muscles that abduct the shoulder on one side—
isotonic work—and those that extend the arm
on the other—isometric work.*
Starting Position: *Stand, hands at left hip level, elbows straight, holding
the ends of an eighteen-inch exercise band.*
How To Do the Exercise: *Stretch the exercise band by moving the right arm
up and away, with thumb pointing to the ceiling while left arm remains
fixed at left hip level. Then return slowly to starting position.
Repeat five to ten times, progressing to fifteen repetitions.
Switch sides and repeat.*
What To Watch For: *Proceed as in previous exercises (see information
regarding Figure 11.11).*

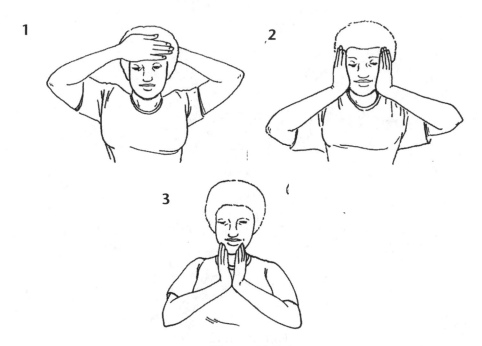

Figure 11.14
Muscle Groups Involved: Muscles that control the movements of the head and neck. Isometric work.
Starting Position: Stand or sit in front of a mirror. **Position 1:** *Place one hand on forehead, the other at the back of head.* **Position 2:** *Place one hand on one side of head, the other on the other side.* **Position 3:** *Place right fingers on right side of chin and the left fingers on the other side.*
How To Do the Exercise: Position 1: *Keeping the hands against the head, press your head against one hand and then the other without moving either your head or your hands. Do not relax tension between presses.*
Position 2: *Keeping your hands against your head, press your head against one hand and then the other without moving either your head or your hands. Do not relax tension between presses.* **Position 3:** *Without turning your chin to left or right, press your chin against the fingers of one hand and then the other. Do not relax tension between presses.*
What To Watch For: *If you have neck pain, start positions 2 and 3 lying on your back. Gradually build up the presses so that contractions are smooth and flow from hand to hand without moving your head. If you have inflammatory arthritis in your upper spine, do not attempt these exercises without professional supervision.*

Looking Forward

The greatest challenge for patients with arthritis is figuring out how to fit an exercise program into their daily lives and adhere to it faithfully and consistently. You are the only one who has the power to make your life better with exercise. Take the first step to wellness today and get started on a muscle-strengthening regime. It can make a real difference in terms of increased mobility and decreased pain if you do it right and stick to it. The following chapter offers additional exercise information designed to help you improve your fitness and endurance.

Chapter 12

Improving Fitness and Endurance

Physical fitness is to the human body what fine-tuning is to an engine. It helps us to perform to our potential. Being fit equates with being in a condition that helps us look, feel, and function at our best. According to the National Institutes of Health: "Fitness is the ability to perform daily tasks in a vigorous and alert manner, with energy left over for enjoying leisure-time activities and meeting emergency needs. It helps us endure, bear up, tolerate stress and carry on, where an unfit person could not continue, and is a major basis for good health and well-being."

Physical fitness involves the performance of the heart, the lungs, and the skeletal muscles. And, since what we do with our bodies affects what we can do with our minds, fitness also involves our intellect and emotions. Fitness promotes alertness and emotional stability. Fitness and health are individual qualities that vary among people. Fitness is influenced by gender, heredity, personal habits, exercise, and eating practices. You have full control over personal habits, exercise, and what you eat and drink. These factors—all of which you are able to control—determine whether you become and stay fit.

In this chapter, we explain the importance of fitness and provide information on getting started with a cardiovascular exercise program to complement the flexibility and muscular strength and endurance exercises you learned about in Chapters 10 and 11.

WHY IS FITNESS IMPORTANT FOR ME?

Physical fitness programs originated in the field of exercise science and originally involved only healthy, athletic young men. The goal of these early programs was to improve the competitive performance in individuals who were already fit by using intense exercise programs. In the past three decades, the importance of physical fitness programs to ordinary people who may be unfit, or those who suffer from chronic diseases such as arthritis, has been recognized.

Among people with arthritis, the pain that results from joint inflammation or degeneration can be very disabling and may cause prolonged inactivity. This prolonged inactivity can, in turn, add dramatically to pain, stiffness, weakness, functional limitations, and disabilities.   The major organ involvement seen in rheumatoid arthritis and lupus can also lead to severe disability and poor physical performance, because these systemic forms of arthritis can affect the heart, lungs, kidneys, and liver, and the gastrointestinal and urinary systems.

It is not necessary for people with arthritis to participate in intensive fitness programs to improve their general health. Moderate physical activities performed on a regular basis can greatly benefit people who are unfit or who suffer from chronic diseases. A total of thirty minutes per day of moderately intense physical activity such as walking or household chores, dispersed throughout the day, can maintain and significantly improve general health.

A regular exercise fitness program has been proven to:

+ Strengthen the heart and cardiovascular system.

+ Improve circulation and help the body utilize oxygen, deliver nutrition to tissues, and remove tissue waste products.

+ Increase energy and activity levels so that more physical work can be done before you get tired.

+ Increase tolerance to pain through the action of the body's own opiates.

+ Increase muscular strength and endurance.

+ Lower blood pressure.

+ Improve balance and joint flexibility.

+ Improve the nutrition of joint cartilage.

+ Strengthen the structure of bones.

+ Improve self-image and self-esteem.

+ Reduce stress, tension, anxiety, and depression.

+ Reduce body fat and help you attain and maintain a healthy body weight.

+ Improve lovemaking and sleep.

+ Help with rest and relaxation.

+ Promote a feeling of fitness and health.

HOW DO I PREPARE
FOR A FITNESS PROGRAM?

If you are younger than thirty-five years of age and are bothered by osteoarthritis in just one or two joints, or if you have another mild form of arthritis, you don't need to see a physician before beginning an exercise program. In a non-medical setting, such as a local gym, you may be asked to complete the Physical Activity Readiness Questionnaire, also known as PAR-Q (Figure 12.1 on the next page). The PAR-Q is often used for initial screening before exercise testing is done or before you begin an exercise fitness program.

If you are older than thirty-five years of age and have a mild form of arthritis, consult a physician who may or may not recommend a graded exercise test. He or she may also perform a general medical workup to look for the following conditions:

✦ High blood pressure.

✦ Heart trouble.

✦ Family history of early stroke or heart-attack deaths.

✦ Frequent dizzy spells.

✦ Extreme breathlessness after mild exertion.

✦ Other known or suspected disease.

These symptoms do not exclude you from a fitness program, but they do indicate the need for vigilance in self-monitoring and participating in a fitness program that is also carefully monitored by your physician, a physical therapist, or a fitness specialist.

PAR-Q PHYSICAL ACTIVITY READINESS QUESTIONNAIRE

For most people, physical activity should not pose any problem or hazard. PAR-Q has been designed to identify the small number of adults for whom physical activity might be inappropriate or those who should have medical advice concerning the type of activity most suitable for them.

Common sense is your best guide in answering these few questions. Please read them carefully and check the "yes" or "no" opposite the question if it applies to you.

	YES	NO	QUESTION
1.	___	___	Has your doctor ever said you have heart trouble?
2.	___	___	Do you frequently have pains in your heart and chest?
3.	___	___	Do you often feel faint or have spells of severe dizziness?
4.	___	___	Has a doctor ever said your blood pressure was too high?
5.	___	___	Has your doctor ever told you that you have a bone or joint problem such as arthritis that has been aggravated by exercise, or might be made worse with exercise?
6.	___	___	Is there a good physical reason not mentioned here why you should not follow an activity program even if you wanted to?
7.	___	___	Are you over age 65 and not accustomed to vigorous exercise?

If you answered YES to one or more questions . . .
If you have not recently done so, consult with your personal physician by telephone or in person before increasing your physical activity and/or taking a fitness test.

If you answered NO to all questions . . .
If you answered PAR-Q accurately, you have reasonable assurance of your present suitability for exercise.

Figure 12.1
You may be asked to fill out a PAR-Q before undergoing exercise testing or beginning an exercise fitness program.

**Most people with arthritis should not begin
a fitness program without first consulting a physician,
rheumatologist, or physical therapist.**

If you have moderate or advanced systemic arthritis, such as rheumatoid arthritis, you should be under the care of your family physician or a rheumatologist if you plan to exercise. You can expect to receive the same medical workup discussed above and, if your physician deems it necessary, a graded exercise test.

HOW IS FITNESS ASSESSED?

Fitness is generally assessed in terms of cardiovascular fitness, muscular strength and endurance, and flexibility. Your overall fitness is also affected by your body mass index and your heart rate. In the following material, these terms are defined and explained.

Cardiovascular Fitness

Cardiovascular fitness can be assessed by means of the Graded Exercise Test, also referred to as an *exercise stress test*. This test provides information about how the heart responds to stress. It is done to determine whether there is adequate blood flow to the heart during increased levels of activity. An exercise stress test usually involves walking on a treadmill or pedaling a stationary bike while your electrocardiogram (ECG), heart rate, and blood pressure are monitored. Measurements will be taken before, during, and after the exercise session. It is normal for your heart rate, blood pressure, and breathing rate to increase during the test. During the test, laboratory personnel will ask if you have chest, arm, or jaw pain; shortness of breath or dizziness; lightheadedness; or any other unusual symptoms. These symptoms should be reported immediately.

Patients with advanced arthritis of lower limb joints and the potential for cardiovascular or pulmonary problems must have a careful medical history and medical review performed before any marked increase in physical activity is prescribed. In this case, a more rigorous test, called a submaximal or symptom-limited stress test, may be required. Ask your physician if you believe you may be a candidate for this type of test.

Cardiovascular fitness can be enhanced by aerobic exercise—physical conditioning designed to enhance circulatory and respiratory efficiency and thus increase the body's oxygen consumption. Aerobic exercise often involves vigorous, sustained exercise, such as walking fast, dancing, swimming, or bicycling. At the end of this chapter, we provide more information about forms of aerobic exercise appropriate for people with arthritis.

Muscular Strength and Endurance

The capacity of a muscle to sustain contractions over a period of time determines its fitness. This capacity is tested with timed movement repetitions at submaximal effort. The higher the number of repetitions within a given time period, the higher the muscular endurance. Measurements used to test endurance include distance walked, number of steps climbed, or the number of laps completed in a swimming pool. The number of activities you can complete over a given period of time is the basis for assessment. Muscular strength and endurance can be improved by the exercises provided in Chapter 11.

Flexibility

The ability of a joint or a related structure to carry out an active movement, or of a muscle group to stretch or extend to the greatest length possible, is an indication of flexibility. In patients with arthritis, the combination of the disease process, inactivity, and pain produce decreased range of motion, stiffness, and general inflexibility in a joint. It is important that stiff joints and tight muscles be warmed up with flexibility exercises and stretches before you begin an endurance exercise session. Flexibility can be improved by engaging in the exercises described in Chapter 10.

Body Mass

The proportion of lean body mass to fat body mass is a better way to evaluate obesity than body weight alone. The fat body mass in men should not exceed 20 percent, and in women, it should be 30 percent or less. Body-fat content can be assessed by measuring skin folds and waist/hip girth ratios. Other more complicated techniques for assessing body fat that can be administered by fitness experts include underwater weighing tanks that measure displacement and sophisticated, computerized systems that measure resistance to the passage of an electrical current through the body.

Another way to assess weight is to calculate the body mass index, or BMI. The body mass index is based on height and weight and applies to both men and women. The BMI can be considered an alternative for direct measures of body fat. It is an inexpensive and easy-to-perform method of screening for weight categories that may lead to health problems. However, the BMI is not a diagnostic tool. A person can have a high BMI, but that alone would not indicate that he or she is unfit or overweight. To really determine if excess weight is a health risk, a health-care provider needs to perform further assessments.

With the metric system, the formula for the BMI is weight in kilograms (kg) divided by height in meters (m) squared. If you are more familiar with pounds and inches, calculate the BMI by dividing your weight in pounds (lbs) by your height in inches (in) squared, and multiplying by a conversion factor of 703. Alternatively, you can find numerous BMI calculators on the Internet to do the math for you. Table 12.1 lists the BMI categories.

If you have a high body-fat percentage or BMI, you may want to consider a weight-management program if your health-care team thinks it is a good idea. Effective weight-management programs emphasize both a healthy diet and physical exercise, which increases muscle bulk and stimulates the burning of fat by expending energy, thereby reducing body fat.

Table 12.1
BMI Categories

- Underweight = <18.5
- Normal weight = 18.5–24.9
- Overweight = 25–29.9
- Obesity = BMI of 30 or greater

A BALANCED WORKOUT

A workout schedule for an exercise fitness program should consist of three parts: a warm-up; exercise to increase muscle strength, endurance, and aerobic capacity; and a cool-down. How often, how long, and how hard you exercise, and what kinds of aerobic exercise you do, should be determined by what condition you are currently in and what your goals are. Your present fitness level, age, health, skills, interests, and convenience are among the factors you should take into account. Obviously, an athlete training for high-level competition would follow a different program than a person with arthritis whose goals are good health and the ability to meet work and recreational needs. Develop your workout goals accordingly.

Warming up and cooling down help prevent injury.

Your exercise fitness program should include something to address each of the following four basic fitness components: flexibility, muscular strength, muscular endurance, and cardiovascular endurance. Flexibility and muscular strength and endurance have been covered in Chapters 10 and 11. The end of this chapter contains more information about improving your cardiovascular endurance with aerobic exercise. Each workout should begin with a warm-up and end with a cool-down. As a general rule, space workouts throughout the week and avoid consecutive days of hard exercise. It is recommended that the average person with arthritis meet the following requirements each week: five to ten minutes of warm-up per each exercise session; two twenty-minute sessions of muscular strength training; two twenty-minute sessions of muscular endurance exercise; three twenty-minute sessions of cardiovascular endurance (aerobic exercise); five to ten minutes of cool down after each exercise session.

The Importance of Warming Up

It is essential that you warm up before beginning your exercise program. It prepares your muscles, joints, and cardiovascular system for your chosen targeted exercise program. A targeted program may consist of muscle strengthening, muscular endurance, or a cardiovascular component. During the warm-up, exercises are done to improve joint movements, make muscles and joints more flexible, and prepare the body for more vigorous activity. Warming up helps you to exercise safely and avoid injuries that could result from the exercise. This is particularly important for patients with arthritis. Your warm-up can be as simple as five to ten minutes of walking, and doing arm circles and trunk rotations. The movements should be low intensity and simulate the movements you will use in your subsequent exercise session. It may also be helpful to precede a warm-up session with a hot shower. Other ideas for warm-up exercises can be found in Chapter 10.

The Importance of Muscular Strength and Endurance

Muscle strengthening using resistance training has been covered in detail, along with muscular endurance exercise, in Chapter 11. Increasing and maintaining the strength of your muscles is an important part of good health and fitness. The benefits of this type of exercise apply to people of all ages and all conditions. Even individuals in their seventies and eighties can increase muscle bulk and decrease body fat with regular muscle strengthening exercise.

Anyone at any age can benefit from engaging in some form of exercise.

Muscular endurance exercises at low intensity and high repetition rates can include push-ups, sit-ups, or pull-ups modified for use by arthritis patients, as well as weight training for all the major muscle groups.

The Importance of Cardiovascular Exercise

The cardiovascular component of your exercise program should consist of continuous aerobic rhythmic exercise. Popular aerobic-conditioning activities include brisk walking, jogging, swimming (water aerobics), rowing, and cross-country skiing. At the end of this chapter, more details are provided to help you choose and get started with an aerobic activity that is right for you.

Cardiovascular conditioning improves heart, lung, and muscle function. Aerobic activities increase stamina by improving oxygen consumption of the muscles.

Some activities can be used to fulfill more than one of your basic exercise requirements. For example, in addition to increasing cardiovascular endurance, walking builds muscular endurance in the legs, and swimming develops the arm, shoulder, and chest muscles. If you select the proper activities, it is possible to fit parts of your muscular endurance workout into your cardiovascular workout and save time. The type of exercise you choose should not exceed your endurance limits. Moderation here is the key word. The advice of your therapist or an exercise expert will be helpful and can alert you to the dos and don'ts of your current health status.

Basic Exercise Principles

The keys to selecting the right kinds of exercises in order to develop and maintain each of the basic components of fitness are found in these principles:

+ The exercise program you choose should be specific to the kind of activity in which you are interested. For example, to do well in swimming, the muscles involved in swimming need to be trained for the movements required. It doesn't necessarily follow that a good jogger is a good swimmer.

+ Include time for play, work, and exercise every day. Remember that exercise needs to be a priority in your life. If you can combine your exercise time with your playtime, it can become more interesting and fun.

+ Exercise hard enough, at levels that are vigorous for long enough periods, to bring about improvement. Strive for stress without distress.

+ You can't hoard physical fitness. Work out regularly in order to keep your body in shape.

+ Increase the intensity, frequency, or duration of activity over a period of time in order to continue reaping benefits.

+ Give your body a chance to adjust to a new routine.

+ Don't get discouraged if you don't see immediate results.

+ Don't give up if you miss a day; just get back on track the following day.

+ Find a partner for a little motivation and socialization.

+ If you are exercising regularly, build some rest periods into your day and some rest days into your weekly exercise schedule.

+ Listen to your body. If you have difficulty breathing or experience faintness or fatigue during or after exercise, consult your physician.

If your joints are painful and swollen two hours after an exercise session, it is an indication that you have gone too far and should reduce the exercise intensity for the next session.

What Can My Heart Rate Tell Me?

Heart-rate monitoring during and after jogging, swimming, cycling, and other aerobic activities is widely accepted as a good method for measuring exercise intensity. Exercise that raises your heart rate to a certain level and keeps it there for twenty minutes can contribute significantly to cardiovascular fitness. This is also referred to as aerobic exercise. You should discuss an appropriate heart-rate target range with your health-care team and fitness instructors in order to raise it and maintain it at the required level, taking into account your age and physical condition.

What Should I Wear When I Exercise?

When you exercise, wear loose-fitting clothing to permit freedom of movement and help you feel comfortable and self-assured. As a general rule, wear lighter clothing than temperatures might indicate. Exercise generates great amounts of body heat. Light-colored clothing that reflects the sun's rays is cooler in the summer. When the weather is very cold, it is better to wear several layers of light clothing than one or two heavy layers. The extra layers help trap heat, and it is easy to shed a layer or two if you become too warm.

In cold weather and in hot sunny weather, it is a good idea to wear something on your head. Ski caps are recommended in the winter; some form of tennis hat or baseball cap that provides shade and can be soaked in water is good in the summer. Never wear rubberized or plastic clothing, as it interferes with the evaporation of perspiration and causes your body temperature to rise to a dangerous level.

The most important item of equipment for the walker is a pair of sturdy, properly fitting walking or running shoes with heavy, cushioned soles, arch supports, and a firm heel cup.

When Should I Exercise?

Among the factors you should consider when establishing a time to work out are your job, your family responsibilities, the availability of exercise facilities, the weather, and your personal preferences. It is important to schedule your workouts at a time when there is little chance that you will have to cancel or interrupt them due to other demands on your time.

The hour just before the evening meal is a popular time for exercise. It provides a welcome change of pace at the end of the day and helps dissolve the day's worries and tensions. Another popular time is early morning, before the workday starts, if your morning pain and discomfort levels allow for this. Those who exercise in the morning say that it makes them more alert and energetic on the job. And you have less chance of getting behind in your schedule and skipping a workout if you do it first thing in the morning.

Studies show that morning exercisers are less likely to skip a workout schedule.

Do not exercise strenuously during extremely hot, humid weather or within two hours after eating a full meal. Heat and digestion both make heavy demands on the circulatory system and, in combination with exercise, can overtax your body.

RECOMMENDED AEROBIC WORKOUTS

There are numerous ways to improve your cardiovascular endurance and aerobic performance, but not all are well suited to the needs of patients with arthritis. The activities that are commonly recommended are walking, water aerobics, and bicycling.

Walking

Walking is one of the easiest ways to improve your cardiovascular performance. It does not require any special equipment except good supportive shoes, appropriate clothing, and, in some cases, a cane. Walking, unlike jogging, is easy on your joints and requires no special skills. Nordic walking—simulating cross-country skiing on dry land—has become very popular. It is kind to your joints and provides a workout for upper and lower limbs; all that is needed is a pair of specially designed "skiing" poles.

Walking requires no special skills or equipment and can be done almost anywhere.

It is easy to custom-tailor walking programs; you can walk as long as you want, as quickly as you want, and where you want. How far and how long you can walk depend on your ability and previous walking experience. Walking one to three miles, three times a week, takes little time and can make you feel and look better. Give yourself a chance to build up and gradually increase your distance and duration. Start with ten minutes and gradually increase your time to between thirty and forty-five minutes. When you reach forty-five minutes, pick up the pace and walk faster until you can cover three miles in forty-five minutes.

Water Exercise

Unlike aerobics on dry land, aerobic exercise in water is easy on your joints, and you do not have to be able to swim a stroke to do water exercises in shallow water.

The following are some key things to remember about water exercises:

+ The buoyancy of the water supports your body and eases the stress on your lower limb joints. Only 10 percent of your body weight is resting on your joints if you stand in shoulder-high water.

+ It is easier to move your joints as they float upward in the water. Pressing your limbs down against the water's buoyancy can offer twelve times more resistance than air and can help strengthen your muscles. The faster you press down, the greater the resistance.

+ Warm water is soothing and a great stress reliever. And the pressure it exerts on your legs can aid circulation. For arthritis patients, a water temperature of eighty-four to eighty-eight degrees Fahrenheit (29 to 31 degrees Celsius) is recommended, with an absolute minimum of eighty-three degrees Fahrenheit (28 degrees Celsius).

+ Water keeps your body aligned in a proper workout position.

+ Because water exercises are easy to do, you may be tempted to do more than you are capable of doing. Do not overdo it, and start slowly. Respect your limitations.

+ Do warm-up and cool-down exercises when you are exercising in the water, just as you would do for land activities.

+ The main session should consist of continuous aerobic activity in which you maintain an exertion level that allows you to keep your breathing under control. Intersperse exercises with short rest intervals.

✦ As you become more comfortable with the exercises, work more powerfully against the water's resistance.

✦ Be careful, and stay behind the point of pain, nudging the level of intensity in each succeeding session.

Exercises that you can do in shallow, waist- or chest-deep water include walking, bending your knees, swinging your legs sideways, and letting your arms float upward. In deep water, a flotation device can keep your head above water and your body upright. Moving your legs to simulate jumping, jogging, cross-country skiing, or cycling motions in the pool can be beneficial exercises. Keep in mind that these put more demand on your cardiovascular system than exercise in shallow water and should not be overdone.

**Exercising in water is a great way
to become more active.**

Other water exercises that are gentle on your joints include water aerobic classes as well as lap swimming. For people with moderate to severe arthritis, exercising in water may be the best way to start becoming more active.

Bicycling

Riding a stationary bike or a real bike can be a good alternative to swimming and walking. If your joints are stable and you can maintain your balance, riding a bike in the fresh air is often more fun than using a stationary bicycle. The same rules regarding warm-up and cool-down exercises apply for biking just as they do for swimming and walking.

Riding a well-fitted bicycle is important. The pedals must allow each leg to straighten completely on the downward swing, with the ball of the foot resting on the pedal. Your arms should be slightly bent at the elbow when you are gripping and holding the handlebars. Your back should be slightly bent in a relaxed and comfortable position. When you bike, stay behind the point of pain, nudging the level of intensity on succeeding rides.

Looking Forward

Whether you choose to walk, swim, bike, or enjoy a different activity, aerobic exercise can do wonders for how you feel, both physically and mentally. Combining cardiovascular exercise with muscular strength and endurance training and flexibility workouts will allow you to do more and feel better every day. This chapter introduced you to the benefits and basic how-tos of aerobic exercise. In the next chapter, you can look forward to more how-tos about protecting your joints and conserving your energy.

Chapter 13

Protecting Joints and Conserving Energy

The previous chapters gave you the knowledge you need to be as fit as you can be. Fitness is important when you have arthritis because it can help keep you strong and energetic. Energy is crucial to feeling good and living well. In addition to getting and staying fit, it makes sense to do all that you can in your daily life to protect yourself from injury and keep your energy levels high. This chapter offers suggestions for ways in which you can carry out your daily activities while protecting your joints from unnecessary stress and strain and saving your energy.

Swollen, tender joints can make even the simplest activity a challenge. Just the notion of dressing, washing, or preparing meals can become disheartening. One of the best ways to adjust to the changes in your life is to learn which tools can help you more easily accomplish tasks while you protect your joints at the same time.

There are dozens of strategies you can employ to take good care of your joints and make the most of your limited supply of energy. Practicing the dual principles of joint protection and energy conservation can help you manage pain, maintain your independence, reduce disability, and improve the quality of your life.

HOW CAN I PROTECT MY JOINTS?

Joints that are inflamed or damaged are more at risk from the stresses of everyday activities. People with arthritis often need to learn how to protect their joints from these stresses by changing the ways in which they carry out certain tasks. This may involve using devices that take the strain off of joints, wearing splints that support joints, or using better body mechanics.

Doing things differently or employing devices with which you are not familiar is not always easy. It can be difficult to change your routines and habits, but if you take the time to analyze the activities that you carry out each day and do some problem-solving around the tasks that you identify as difficult, you can surprise yourself with how much you can accomplish by modifying your approach.

As you think about changes that you can make, think honestly about what you like to do, what you need to do, and what you can eliminate. For example, if you enjoy baking but find stirring difficult, you could use a food processor. Do you really need to stand while you do ironing, or could you do it while sitting? You may want to continue to be in charge of meal preparation, but can somebody else carry in the groceries and put them away?

Ask yourself, "What do I like to do, what do I need to do, and what can I eliminate?"

HOW CAN I CONSERVE MY ENERGY?

Arthritis can rob you of energy in a number of ways. If you have inflammatory arthritis, fatigue can be one of the systemic features of your condition, making you wonder if you can make it through the next small task. If your muscles have become weakened and your movement is impaired, you will find yourself working at a biomechanical disadvantage. It may take more of your energy to rise from a chair and walk across the room than it would if your joints and muscles were in good shape.

**Remember to plan in advance, which will
save you energy in the long run.**

Think of yourself as having a "savings account" of energy. You have only so much energy to last until you can rest and deposit more energy into your account. You do not want to spend all that energy at one time or in one place. Just as people need regular deposits in their bank accounts, people with arthritis need to make regular deposits of rest into their energy account.

Because sleep at night may be disturbed as a result of pain, many people with arthritis say that they are still tired when they wake up in the morning. If this happens to you, ask your doctor about using pain medication or a muscle relaxant at night to help you sleep better. In this way, you can avoid starting the day with an energy deficit.

Save your energy! It's like money in the bank.

HOW CAN I MANAGE
INDEPENDENTLY AT HOME?

At home, people with arthritis encounter challenges in everyday activities such as bathing, toileting, brushing teeth and hair, preparing meals, doing laundry, and cleaning. The home is also probably the place in which you conduct the majority of your leisure activities.

If you have problems with hand function, standing from a sitting position, walking, climbing stairs, reaching shelves, or bending to pick up objects, you may feel that the barriers to independent living are almost insurmountable. To make your life easier, you're probably going to need to make some changes, and you may need some help along the way.

How Can an Occupational Therapist Help Me?

Spending some time with an occupational therapist (OT) who is experienced in the needs of arthritis patients can pay great dividends. Research evidence indicates that occupational therapy helps people to accomplish tasks such as dressing, cooking, and cleaning.

**OTs can show you how to protect
your joints and pace yourself.**

OTs have special skills in problem-solving; they can help you plan your work schedule so that you can prioritize activities and pace yourself. They can also teach you how to properly position your joints as you work and rest. They can recommend assistive devices, suggest adaptations to your home or work setting, advise you on proper footwear, and prescribe or have splints custom-made to protect inflamed or unstable joints.

Principles of Joint Protection

OTs can train you and advise you about joint protection. The following principles can help you decide what things you can change, what you can stop doing, or what you can do differently.

+ Respect your pain. Pain exists to tell you to stop, slow down, shorten the time of the activity, change the way you do it, or get help.

+ Change your position often. Holding joints in one position for a long time can increase pain and fatigue.

+ Take frequent breaks. Avoid doing one task over a long period. Stand up, stretch, and relax. Break the job down into smaller pieces.

+ Rely on your largest, strongest joints and muscles. Carry your handbag over your shoulder instead of in your hand. Instead of pushing a door open with your hand, use your shoulder or hip.

+ Maintain good posture and positioning. Poor posture robs you of energy because your joints are not aligned properly.

+ Alternate heavy jobs with lighter tasks. If you are cleaning the bathroom, take a break and fold some laundry. A change of activity is a form of rest for overused joints and muscles.

+ Use the best tools for the job. Assistive devices, large handles, levers, and wrist and hand splints all reduce strain on affected joints.

✦ Maintain your strength, mobility, and endurance. Your exercise program is important in maintaining your independence.

Choosing the Right Tools

Arthritis can affect individuals differently, depending on the type and severity of the disease. An assistive device (tool) that is suitable for one person may not be suitable for another. Advice from an occupational therapist can be invaluable in helping you choose the right tools for the tasks that you want or need to do. Think about the tasks that you regularly find difficult and that you may not be able to do independently. Ask yourself the following questions before you purchase an assistive device:

✦ Is the product safe to use?

✦ Is it easy to use? Is it easy to grasp and easy to open and close?

✦ Is it lightweight?

✦ Does it require regular maintenance?

✦ Does it have a textured surface, making it easier to grasp?

✦ Is it worth the expense, or would another product do the job just as well?

Considering these questions will help you avoid cluttering your life with gadgets for which you find no use. For example, an item that might not be a good investment is an electric can opener that takes up counter space and requires significant hand dexterity to use. If at all possible, try out such convenience items before purchasing them.

Work smart not hard!

Many of your daily challenges can be resolved easily and inexpensively with some creativity. Until recent years, most assistive devices were available only in places such as medical-supply retailers, but now, department stores, pharmacies, and hardware stores carry a wide range of products that are relatively inexpensive and easy to use. Some examples are kitchen utensils with large, textured handles, double-handed pots for easy lifting, jar openers, levered tap or door handles, rubberized mats for stabilizing bowls, and even pipe insulation that comes in different sizes and can be cut into short lengths to fit over cutlery, pencils, toothbrushes, etc. Examples of some of these devices are illustrated in Figures 13.1 through 3.3.

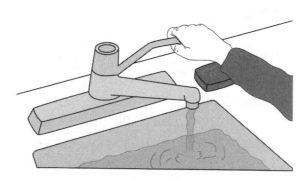

Figure 13.1
Levered taps are easier to use than other types of handles.

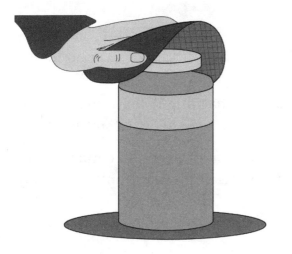

Figure 13.2
A rubberized material can help you to grip jar lids.

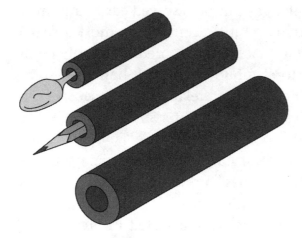

Figure 13.3
*Pipe insulation can be used
to enlarge handles.*

Tips to Get The Day Started Right

Arthritis pain is often worse in the morning. When you wake up, you may wonder how on earth you will be able to open the pill bottle, hold your toothbrush, take a shower, reach up to brush your hair, and make it into your clothes. Don't be discouraged. Instead, make an effort to start each day in a healthy way—do your range-of motion-exercises and a few stretches (see Chapter 10). Follow them with a warm shower.

Start the day off right!

Here is some additional advice that might help you make it through your morning routine with more energy to spare:

✦ Ask your pharmacist to provide easy-to-open pill containers, or store your pills in a dosette, a container that holds your daily dose of medication for each day of the week.

- ✦ Consider buying a lightweight electric toothbrush with a wide handle.

- ✦ Purchase a sling towel that has loops at either end. You can find this in medical-supply stores and in some pharmacies.

- ✦ Buy a hairbrush with a long, padded handle, which is easier to maneuver.

- ✦ A dressing stick, with rubber-coated hooks at either end, can help you pull on socks, lift bra straps, and adjust sleeves in garments.

- ✦ Elastic shoelaces and a long-handled shoehorn can help with putting on shoes.

- ✦ Buy clothing such as tops, blouses, pants, and bras with front closures. Velcro, large buttons, or buttonhooks are good choices.

- ✦ Put a loop of tape or a key ring through the top of zippers to make pulling easier.

If you don't struggle through the first steps of the day, you can save your energy for the things that you really need and want to do.

PUT SAFETY FIRST

Safety is an important concern when you have arthritis. Limited mobility and weak muscles can put you at risk of a fall, which could have serious consequences. Check your home for loose carpets that may slide under your foot, or telephone or electrical cords that could cause you to trip. Rid your home of clutter! Make sure that stairwells and hallways are unobstructed and well lit and that you have a nightlight in the bathroom.

Set up your living space so that you can safely rise from chairs and sofas without needing to reach out for assistance. Getting up by grabbing a piece of furniture is dangerous, because furniture may give way or move. You can raise the height of a chair by putting it up on a platform or on blocks (Figure 13.4). Another simple solution is to add a raised cushion covered in a nonslip fabric to chairs and sofas. These cushions are commercially available and are lightweight; often they have a strap attached so that they can be carried from place to place (Figure 13.5). These can be a great help if you are riding in a car, going to the movies, or are out visiting.

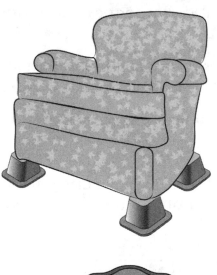

Figure 13.4
Raise the height of your seating.

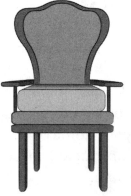

Figure 13.5
A raised cushion can be taken
with you.

Make sure that your stairs have railings to provide support and that the stair treads have nonslip surfaces. Do not place loose carpets at the top or bottom of a staircase, and be sure that the stairwell is clearly lit. Try to limit the numbers of trips you need to make up and down stairs. Keep a basket or bag handy to collect items that you wish to take from one floor to another. Problem-solve and be creative to make your life easier. You can even put laundry in a pillowcase and toss it downstairs if your laundry room is on a lower level!

Being safe is being smart.

If walking is difficult or painful due to pain or deformity, particularly in the hips and knees, a cane can reduce the stress through the painful joint by as much as 50 percent. It can also contribute to your safety, because if a joint is painful or unstable, you are much more likely to have a fall. Use the cane in the hand that is on the opposite side from the most painful joint. Be sure to have the cane measured for correct length. When you hold the cane by your side and slightly away from your foot, make sure that the handle is level with the crease of your wrist. The cane should have a good, solid, rubber tip. For the winter months, you can purchase a retractable ice pick for the tip. Canes come in a variety of shapes and are available with contoured handles (rather than inverted, U-shaped handles), which make them easier to use if you have arthritis in your hands (Figure 13.6).

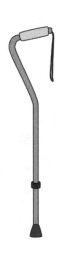

Figure 13.6
A cane can reduce pain and make you more safe.

If walking outdoors or in a shopping mall is difficult, or if you need to carry parcels, a wheeled walker with a basket and a fold-down seat is a good idea, because you can rest wherever you are and your hands are spared the stress of carrying items.

Avoid heavy lifting, especially if you have arthritis that affects your back. If you must lift something, face the object squarely, bend your knees, and use the muscles of your legs. Hold the object close to your body. Pushing or sliding heavy objects is preferable, as is using a dolly or cart. See Figures 13.7 and 13.8 for ideas on how to move objects efficiently.

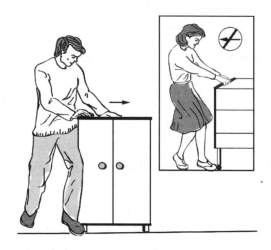

Figure 13.7
Push, don't pull!

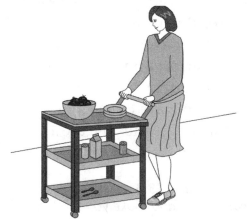

Figure 13.8
Use a wheeled cart to save time and energy.

Bathroom Safety

Most accidents in the home occur in the bathroom, which is not surprising considering the obstacles (wet surfaces, a low toilet, and the difficulty presented by getting in and out of the bathtub). To ensure safety, make sure that your bathmat has a rubberized back and that the bathtub has a nonslip mat or decals. It is wise to have an easy-to-grip bar installed on the side of the bathtub and another on the nearby wall. Medical-supply retailers sell these, and many will install them free of charge.

If you are unable to safely enter and exit the tub, many types of bath benches are available. Some are little more than benches with rubber feet. Others fit into the bathtub and have an extended seat that projects so that you can sit outside the tub and then lift your legs into it (see Figure 13.9). You can try out these benches at the suppliers' store to find out what suits you best.

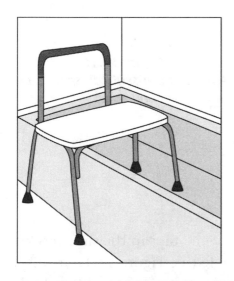

Figure 13.9
This bath bench fits over the side of the tub.

Bath seats are usually used with a handheld shower head. You may want to consider purchasing a new bathtub with a side-door opening for easy entry and exit. A large shower stall that can accommodate two is ideal if you have difficulty getting into a bathtub. The extra size can also be useful if you wish to exercise or need the help of another person to shower. Again, you will need a rubberized mat or a bath seat with rubber tips.

You want to be certain that you can sit on and rise from the toilet without holding onto the sink or the paper dispenser, which can be not only risky but dangerous. A raised toilet seat is invaluable, particularly if you have hip or knee problems. The toilets come in various heights, and some have armrests attached for added safety (see Figure 13.10). Recently, higher toilets have become available for purchase, and you can even buy what is known as a toilet extender, which is installed under the base of the toilet. Both of these are obviously more costly, but they are generally thought to be less obvious in appearance than a raised seat.

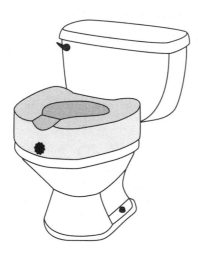

Figure 13.10
A raised toilet seat can spare hips and knees.

To reduce strain on your hands, levered taps in the sink and tub are easy to use and are readily available (see Figure 13.1). If this is not possible, use a gripping device, such as a piece of textured rubber, or a commercial product that fits over your existing taps.

Kitchen Safety

The kitchen is another area of the home in which accidents occur. The first step in eliminating hazards is to organize your work space and storage areas so that you are less at risk for incurring falls, spills, or burns. Organization is the key to safety and to protecting your joints and saving energy. The following suggestions can help you ensure your safety in the kitchen.

✦ Put items that you use frequently within easy reach—on lower shelves, sliding shelves, or lazy Susans.

✦ Consider adding an easy-to-reach shelf between the countertop and cupboard level.

✦ Use a long-handled reacher to grab lightweight items from higher shelves or to reach things in lower cupboards.

✦ To fill a pot with water, place the pot on the stove and add the water gradually with a plastic measuring cup, rather than lugging a heavy, cumbersome, water-filled pot from the sink to the stove.

✦ Choose lightweight pots and pans. When you are transferring a pot from the stove, slide it onto a potholder, then slide the pot and potholder across the counter.

✦ To fill a cup from the kettle, place the cup in the sink and use two hands to tip the kettle over the edge of the sink.

✦ Use a wheeled trolley to transport dishes and cutlery to the table.

✦ Put a looped strap through the refrigerator door. This will allow you to slide your forearm into the loop in order to pull the door open.

✦ Use a high stool on which to sit when you are preparing foods at the counter; alternate between sitting and standing.

✦ When you are stirring or mixing, place the bowl on a rubberized mat or a damp towel and use two hands to stir.

✦ Use utensils that are easy to handle—tools with large, padded grips, jar keys that break the vacuum seals on jar lids, and special lightweight cutting boards that hold vegetables for peeling.

✦ Plan ahead. Think about what kitchen activities you plan to do on a particular day, and ask family or friends to prepare the way by lifting heavy objects, loosening jar lids, opening milk cartons, or getting items out of the freezer.

MAKING LIGHT WORK OF HOUSEWORK

If you have been accustomed to doing all of your own housework and have taken pride in your ability to do so, having arthritis is guaranteed to challenge your skills and require you to think and act differently as you make a priority of looking after your joints and saving your energy. If, on the other hand, you have never particularly enjoyed housework and find it to be drudgery, this is an opportunity to look at ways to eliminate the unnecessary and to simplify household tasks. Whichever camp you fall into, nobody likes to watch the work pile up and become an insurmountable obstacle. There is no better time than now to address the challenges that housework can present.

First, take the time to list the household tasks that you feel *must* be done, daily, weekly, and monthly and ask yourself:

✦ Which tasks are truly necessary? Could any of them be eliminated?

✦ How often do each of these chores really need to be done?

✦ Could any tasks be done less often?

✦ Can you break large jobs down into smaller tasks?

✦ Can you delegate certain jobs to others in the household?

✦ Are your expectations of yourself too high?

✦ Can these tasks be accomplished according to a schedule rather than just by working until they are completed or you are exhausted?

✦ Could a hired housekeeper to do the heavy chores of cleaning, washing clothes, ironing, and vacuuming carpets and floors if these tasks consume a great deal of your energy?

The Five Ps

Once you have answered these questions, you are ready to develop a weekly schedule that allows you to establish a comfortable pace for yourself. You will need to schedule in rest periods with the activities. Remember not to "bunch" too many activities together and to alternate light work with heavier jobs. It also helps to keep the five Ps in mind.

✦ **Plan** your weekly schedule on paper. This will let you see where you could save steps and energy and analyze the priorities.

✦ **Pace** yourself. This is actually a part of the planning. You may not be good at pacing yourself at first; you may need to experiment a little to find what is comfortable for you. Try to follow a tentative schedule for a few weeks, then modify it as you see fit.

✦ **Prioritize** so that you are spending your energy doing the most important tasks. If you find that your expectations have been set too high, ask yourself the questions listed in the previous section again and decide which jobs need to be a priority. While you are setting priorities, remind yourself that rest periods, exercise, and pleasurable activities must be included.

✦ **Position** your joints correctly as you work. This will help you make the most of the energy you have available and will allow you to protect your joints from undue stresses. Proper positioning involves adhering to the principles of joint protection, wearing work splints, using the right tools, and maintaining good posture.

✦ **Problem-solve** with others. Involving family, friends, occupational therapists, and/or your arthritis self-management program (ASMP) group can be a great help. Other people can provide a fresh perspective on your challenges and may have found solutions in their own experiences that can help you.

Cleaning Aids

Cleaning is one of the biggest household chores and certainly the most physically demanding. If you can afford to hire someone to do the cleaning, that is probably the best joint-protection and energy-conservation technique you can follow. If you cannot afford this type of help, look into what resources might be available to you within your community. Ask your doctor or other health-care provider to refer you to the appropriate agency. Some private health-insurance schemes, seniors' programs, and veterans' services cover housekeeping services, or there may be volunteer agencies within your community that could help.

The right tool can help work go faster and easier.

When you must do the cleaning yourself, follow the list below of housecleaning tools and tips that can make your work easier:

✦ Lightweight, battery-operated broom and carpet sweepers, weighing less than four pounds, are inexpensive, so you can keep one on each floor.

✦ Keep a set of cleaning supplies on each floor.

✦ Use long-handled dustpans.

✦ Long-handled, synthetic dusters can extend your reach beyond that of an ordinary dust cloth.

✦ A child's toy mop is great for cleaning bathtubs.

✦ Try a lightweight wet mop with a swivel head for washing floors.

✦ Do smaller loads of wash more frequently.

✦ Purchase easy-care clothing that requires no ironing.

✦ Use a sponge instead of a dishcloth. To remove excess water, push the sponge against the side of the sink to eliminate wringing, which is not good for finger joints.

✦ Let dishes air-dry.

✦ Purchase lightweight products whenever possible.

✦ Use wheels on buckets, garbage cans, and laundry baskets.

✦ Invest in a collapsible shopping cart.

Be creative! Any idea that saves steps or effort is worth trying. If your idea is successful, it is worth sharing with others.

TAKING CARE OF YOUR HANDS

There is almost nothing that you do in the course of a day that doesn't involve the use of your hands, from brushing your teeth to lifting boxes. Some movements of the hands are very fine and require dexterity, such as sewing with a needle, and some are larger movements that require strength, such as gripping a hammer. This section devotes special attention to the care of the many joints in your hands and wrists. These are the joints that are the most vulnerable to stress as you manage your day.

The hands and wrists consist of many joints supported by a large number of tendons lined with synovium and ligaments. (For more information on joint structure, see Chapter 2.) This makes them a target for arthritis. Taking care to preserve the strength and motion in your hands is crucial. In the following content, we describe some ways in which you can do this.

To ease morning stiffness, coat your hands in oil (baby, mineral, or even salad oil), then put on a pair of rubber dishwashing gloves. Soak your hands in water that is as warm as you can tolerate comfortably for five to ten minutes while you bend and stretch your fingers. This procedure provides similar benefits to using a wax bath but is much easier to do and is more economical. You can pack the materials you need to do this and take them with you if you are traveling. You can also do this routine when you are washing dishes.

Avoiding Ulnar Drift

The inflamed joints of the fingers are at risk of damage that can lead to deformity. You can lessen the pain and damage by being aware of how you use your hands. In inflammatory arthritis, the tendency is for the fingers to "drift" from the knuckles toward the little finger. This is called ulnar drift. Try the following strategies to avoid moving your fingers in that direction.

✦ Avoid lifting objects with your fingers alone; curl your hands around objects as you lift them.

✦ Use two hands when you are stirring or lifting articles such as mugs, bowls, or plates (Figure 13.11).

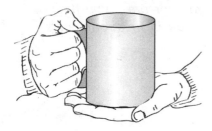

Figure 13.11
Use two hands to hold objects.

✦ Hold handles of utensils, such as brooms, mops, garden tools, etc., straight across your palm (Figure 13.12).

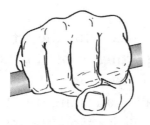

Figure 13.12
Grip handles across the palm.

✦ Don't hold onto things any tighter than you must.

✦ Work toward the middle of your body when you are stirring or wiping surfaces.

✦ Avoid holding things between the pad of your thumb and the side of your index finger.

✦ Use the flat of your palm to open lids; better yet, use a jar-lid opener.

✦ Use your palms or push with the length of your forearms, not the back of your fingers, to get up from a chair (Figure 13.13).

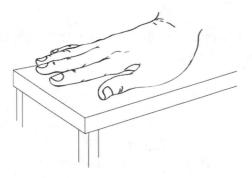

Figure 13.13
Use the flat of your palm or your forearm to push up and avoid stress on fingers.

✦ Relax your hands often and stretch your fingers.

Are Hand Splints Right For Me?

Splints or orthotics (artificial supports or braces) for the wrists, hands, and fingers can be helpful in supporting joints in their proper alignment and in reducing pain and swelling. There are basically two types of splints. The first is called a resting splint or static splint (Figure 13.14); the second is called a working splint (Figure 13.15).

When wrist and finger joints are inflamed and swollen, you want to be sure that you rest them in a good position, particularly at night. Patients report that wearing resting splints can relieve morning stiffness and reduce pain and swelling. A resting splint holds the fingers, the palm, and the wrist, and sometimes the

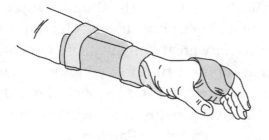

Figure 13.14
Resting splints can relieve
morning stiffness and pain.

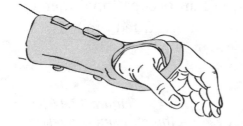

Figure 13.15
A working splint is worn to
protect your joints during
the day.

thumb, in a functional position. Generally, these splints are custom-made by an occupational therapist to ensure that you have a proper fit. If you feel that you would benefit from the use of a resting splint, you should talk with your PT or OT, who can advise you.

A working splint, as its name implies, is worn to protect your joints while you go about your daily activities. Research has shown that these devices can relieve pain and increase strength in the short term and thereby improve the performance of daily activities. However, they may decrease dexterity. These splints come in several forms. Some include the thumb, some have a removable piece of metal or plastic in the palm that can be reshaped to fit the individual hand, and others are custom-made. The important thing here is that the splint fit properly. Always seek professional advice regarding the appropriate type of splint for you. An ill-fitting splint can do more harm than good.

A poorly fitted splint can be harmful.

Osteoarthritis commonly affects the base of the thumb, whose function contributes to pinching and grasping objects. The resulting pain and poor alignment can cause great difficulty. Often, people find that having a splint that supports the affected joint while allowing the thumb to move across the hand and to touch the end of the index finger (Figure 13.16) greatly helps to relieve pain and improve hand function. Thumb splints are available commercially, but you should get the advice of an occupational therapist or an orthotist to make sure that the splint is fitted properly.

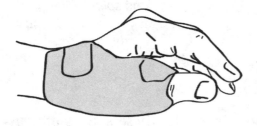

Figure 13.16
A thumb splint can relieve pain and improve hand function.

There are two deformities that can affect the middle joints of the fingers, the *swan-neck* deformity (where the middle joint is hyper-extended) and the *boutonnière* deformity (where the middle joint is hyper-flexed). Both of these can be significantly disabling.

"Ring splints" can be ordered in a variety of metals and can be adjusted to fit the affected joints (Figure 13.17). While there is no evidence that splints actually correct deformities, the use of these splints, if the deformity is not advanced, can assist with function.

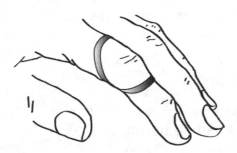

Figure 13.17
Ring splints may assist with function.

At the same time, some consider them to be attractive pieces of jewelry. These must be fitted by someone who is qualified to do so, such as an occupational therapist.

Specially made splints are used following surgical repair of tendon damage or joint replacement. These splints have wires and elastics fitted to them to either assist or resist movement following the operation. They are called dynamic splints and need to be adjusted during the recovery period. Your surgeon will let you know if you are in need of a specialty splint.

TAKING CARE OF YOUR FEET

When your feet hurt, you are likely to limp and develop a poor gait and poor posture. As a result, you may try to avoid walking. If your weight is not distributed evenly on your feet, the rest of your body is in poor alignment, creating stress on your other joints.

Arthritis often results in problems in the joints of the feet. In inflammatory arthritis, the arches of the feet (the long arch from under the ankle to the base of the toes and the arch across the base of the toes) are commonly affected. Deformities such as hammer toes, fallen arches, heel spurs, and many other painful problems can develop.

People with osteoarthritis can develop bunions (a painful enlargement of the joint at the base of the big toe). These problems can be greatly helped by the use of properly fitted shoes and inserts or orthotics (in this case, molded insoles). Think of these as splints for the feet, supporting the joints and arches and taking pressure off of the painful joints.

A shoe that has a low heel, fits firmly around the heel, and supports your arches is best. A good, deep toe box, a flexible sole, and elastic shoelaces are also essential (Figure 13.18). Good running

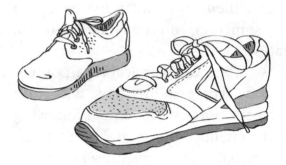

Figure 13.18
Wear properly fitted,
supportive footwear.

shoes are ideal, and several brands have removable insoles so that a custom insole can be substituted. If laces are a problem, some shoes have Velcro closures. You may also want to try elastic shoelaces. Many companies manufacture attractive shoes with all of the qualities listed above. These shoes tend to be more expensive than others, but the return on the investment is great. It is far better to have one or two pairs of properly fitted shoes that allow you to stand and walk in comfort than to have a dozen pairs that are intolerable. It may be tempting to just put on your soft slippers and shuffle along, but this can be very harmful to the feet in the long run.

A pain-free foot makes walking a pleasure.

Remember to do your foot exercises regularly to keep your joints mobile and the small muscles that support them strong. Two examples of easy foot exercises are shown in Figures 13.19 and 13.20.

Consult with an occupational therapist, an orthotist, a podiatrist, or a chiropodist to make sure that you are taking the best possible care of your feet.

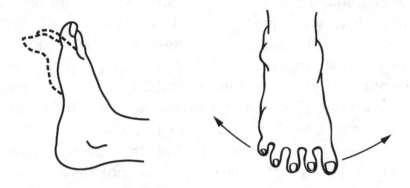

Figure 13.19
*Sitting or lying, bend and stretch your toes as far as
possible. Repeat five times.*

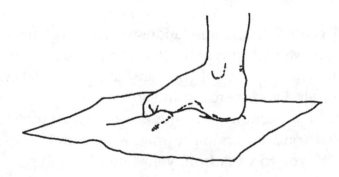

Figure 13.20
*Sitting with your foot on a towel, use your toes to crumple the towel
under your foot. Repeat five times with each foot.*

The skin of the feet can also be affected by inflammatory arthritis. Because your circulation may be affected and pressure points may result from misaligned joints, calluses can form, which cause increased pain. The skin over calluses may break down and become infected. Inspect your feet regularly for reddened skin or discoloration. If you have limited mobility and cannot see the soles of your feet, place a mirror on the floor and hold each foot above the mirror. Wash and dry your feet and the area between your toes carefully to prevent infections from occurring. Devices are available with long handles from some pharmacies and medical supply dealers to help you accomplish foot washing and drying tasks.

HOW CAN I MANAGE INDEPENDENTLY IN THE WORKPLACE?

So far, this chapter has mainly addressed the challenges that may affect a person with arthritis in the home. If you are in the workforce, the same principles apply, but you may have additional challenges.

Ask yourself if you are ready and able to work full-time. Do you need to consider working part-time, or can you arrange for flexible hours so that you are working at times when you feel your best? Is it possible for you to work from your home?

You will need to prioritize your workload and plan ahead for important events, getting more rest at home before spending extra energy. You may need extra time to take breaks. Be sure to use these breaks to rest.

Within your workplace, assess your work space to determine your needs (Figure 13.21). Consider the following questions:

✦ Is your chair comfortable, with armrests and good support for your back?

✦ Do you have a footrest?

✦ Are the items you use regularly within easy reach?

✦ Do you have a computer work surface that allows you to work with your elbows bent at a ninety-degree angle to the keyboard? Do you have proper wrist support?

✦ Do you need to stand for long periods of time?

✦ Could you use a wheeled cart for carrying files or other heavy objects?

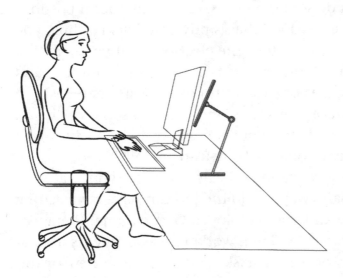

Figure 13.21
Organize your work space and use good posture.

If your job requires you to stand for long periods of time, you may benefit from a sit/stand stool that will allow you to move more easily and change position often. You will also want to wear well-fitted and supportive shoes. Standing on a rubber mat can reduce strain.

**Small, smart changes in your work habits
can make a big difference!**

The ideal chair, if you work at a desk, is adjustable and supports your mid and lower back, your thighs, and your buttocks. Your computer monitor should be about thirty inches from your eyes when you are looking straight ahead. A split keyboard and a trackball mouse will protect your hands and arms from strain. Use a telephone headset to reduce strain on your neck. You should stand up and move around, or do some stretches, every half hour if possible.

If you are employed in a job that is physically demanding, you need to think about safety factors, the positions that you may find difficult, whether your tools are the best for your condition, and how your environment is organized. If possible, alternate tasks to prevent stress on joints and muscles, and take breaks in which you can sit or lie down to replenish your energy. Avoid heavy lifting by pushing or rolling heavy objects or by using a dolly.

Working with the occupational health and safety unit at your work to find easier, safer ways to do the job can have far-reaching benefits both for you and your employer. Occupational therapists can be of great assistance by doing workplace assessments to analyze the components of various tasks and suggesting new or different ways to accomplish work while protecting your joints. In most states and provinces, there are legislated requirements for employers to meet the needs of people with disabilities.

SHOULD I MODIFY MY HOME . . . OR MOVE?

As people with arthritis adjust to the demands of the disease and struggle to maintain their independence, many wonder if it is better to spend a lot of money on home modifications or move to another home that is already more suited to their needs. The answers don't always come easily. Before making this big decision, conduct a survey of your current home and list the barriers that you encounter on a daily basis. Take into account the following:

✦ How many flights of stairs are there, and how often do you use them? Are there railings?

✦ Is the size of the house appropriate for your needs? Do you need fewer rooms to care for?

✦ Are storage spaces, laundry facilities, etc. accessible and easy to use?

✦ Is there sufficient space in the bathroom to be safe? Is the shower opening wide enough and are the taps easy to use?

✦ Is the kitchen well laid out? Are there sufficient cupboards with shelves you can reach?

If you enjoy your house and neighborhood but recognize that some things don't work well for you, it may be that modifications can be made that will address your problems. Railings, door handles, taps, or additional shelves can be installed relatively cheaply. Even the installation of new fixtures such as toilets, bathtubs with side entries, or spacious shower stalls can be well worth the cost. Eliminating stairs is a different proposition, although one alternative is to install a chair lift. Moving laundry facilities from the basement to the first floor can also be costly. If you are planning a renovation, be sure to do your research and get good advice about any architectural changes you consider. Take into account the height of work surfaces. These vary according to individual needs, whether you are short or tall and if you prefer to work standing or sitting. In some states and provinces, government assistance is available for home adaptations, and recommended designs and dimensions can be available. Once again, consulting with an occupational therapist can make it easier for you to develop a plan of action.

Moving to a different house is one of the top ten stressors in a person's life. It should not be undertaken lightly, but it may be that, in the longer term, it is a good decision. If you decide to do so, look into the opportunities of having a house built to your specifications and incorporating some expert advice in advance. Choose a design with easy entry, minimal steps or none at all, with all rooms on one floor. If you have a choice of plumbing fixtures, flooring, doorway width, etc., make the most of it. Having laundry and storage facilities on the same level as the area where you cook, eat, sleep, and bathe makes good sense and will save you energy. Wider hallways and doors makes it easier to navigate in a wheelchair, walker or walking aids. Consider building a linen closet in the bathroom to save extra steps and having ample space in the garage for other main-floor storage options. Remember that planning in advance will save you disappointment and money in the long run.

Looking Forward

This chapter has focused on the things that you can do to save energy and protect your joints while accomplishing daily activities. The following chapter will deal with the ways in which arthritis can affect your emotions and your social relationships and will offer suggestions about maintaining healthy attitudes and relationships.

Chapter 14

Adjusting to the Emotional Impact of Arthritis

Chapter 14 introduces the main causes underlying the emotional changes people often experience when they learn that they have a chronic condition. This chapter is designed to help patients deal with the emotional impact of an arthritis diagnosis and its aftermath. The information in this chapter also can be valuable for spouses, family members, or caregivers of people with arthritis. Whether you are a person with arthritis or someone who cares about a person with arthritis, this chapter will help you to understand the emotional issues surrounding an arthritis diagnosis and assist you in opening lines of communication.

HOW DOES ARTHRITIS AFFECT EMOTIONS?

A diagnosis of systemic arthritis, such as rheumatoid arthritis, can be a big blow to your physical health and well-being, independence,

income, and hopes and plans for the future. People who are diagnosed with arthritis must face the fact that they will experience
pain and discomfort that may be relieved but cannot be cured. A
diagnosis can force a person to make changes in their lifestyle,
relationships, and life roles and possibly to reduce or eliminate certain activities. A study of 197 people with arthritis found that they
were primarily concerned with the following issues:

✦ Worsening of the condition (89 percent).

✦ The chronic nature of the disease, the future, and their ability
   to control the illness (80 percent).

✦ Coping with pain, fatigue, disability, medication side effects,
   and their future financial state (70 to 80 percent).

✦ Family members' lack of understanding of their disease (73 percent).

The concerns of individuals with different types of arthritis were
all similar. With all of that to contend with, it is not surprising that
people become emotionally upset when they find out that they
have arthritis. One of the most common reactions is depression.

**It is natural to feel strong emotions when
you are diagnosed with arthritis.**

Research shows that 13 to 17 percent of people with rheumatoid arthritis show signs of clinical depression in any given year. A
slightly lower percentage of people with osteoarthritis are
depressed. Among people with arthritis, younger people are much
more likely to become depressed than older people. The predictors
of depression are disease activity, disability, and the degree to
which valued activities are affected.

THE GRIEF CYCLE: AN INTRODUCTION

An intense emotional reaction is a normal response when individuals learn that they have a chronic illness like arthritis. This response is very much like the phases of grief described by the well-known psychiatrist, Dr. Elisabeth Kübler-Ross, who documented the effect of grief on people who have experienced the loss of a loved one. In her work, Kübler-Ross described five phases of grieving that are commonly referred to as the "grief cycle." When applied to the reaction to the news that a person has a chronic illness, the phases look something like the following list. In this section, we will introduce the phases; the rest of the chapter is devoted to looking at each phase in the grief cycle in more depth.

1. **Denial.** Nobody wants to hear bad news, and our first reaction to bad news often is to say, "This can't be true. Why should it happen to me? Let's not talk about it. I don't need help, and I am not a member of the group of people who have arthritis!"

2. **Anger.** People can experience anger at family and friends who don't understand and at the medical professionals who can't make the arthritis go away. This may lead to a search for miraculous and unproven cures and/or "shopping" for a doctor who will provide the answers you want to hear.

3. **Bargaining.** People may be inclined to feel that if they were better people, their arthritis would improve. Or they may tell themselves that, if and only if the disease doesn't get worse, they will be able to accept the condition.

4. **Depression.** There are two components to depression: physical and emotional. The physical indicators can be changes in weight or appetite and sleep patterns, difficulty concentrating or making decisions, memory problems, and fatigue or loss of

energy. The emotional signs may include sadness, guilt, worthlessness, hopelessness, irritability, moodiness, excessive crying, loss of interest and/or enjoyment of life, and thoughts of death and even suicide.

5. **Acceptance.** Finally, a person begins to accept the diagnosis, adjust his or her lifestyle accordingly, and become involved in the treatment program. Patients who have accepted their diagnosis choose activities that are appropriate, take good care of themselves, are able to talk about the disease openly, are less focused on the disease, and are able to move forward with their lives.

Understanding the five stages of grieving and learning how to deal with these can help move you forward and allow you to take control of your health. These five stages are normal, although they may not occur in the same sequence. Individuals may even go through one or two stages more than once. Some stages may not last as long as others. If you are experiencing any of these stages, accept them as normal and be encouraged that they don't usually last very long. It is important to know, though, that if depression is not acknowledged and managed in a timely fashion, it may color your life for months and even years. If you feel that you are "stuck" in any one stage, talk to your doctor or social worker about getting help to keep moving through the process.

Denial

For most people, denial is simply a way to soften the blow of the diagnosis. It's an unconscious attempt to avoid the stress or anxiety about loss of independence, pain, and potential lifestyle changes. If denial interferes with accepting the implications of the disease or with getting treatment, it can have serious consequences. Listen carefully to the advice of your health-care team and ask yourself if you are taking a risk by denying that you have a chronic condition. Ignoring the health-care team's advice won't make your condition go away. Sooner or later, your symptoms will force you to face the truth about your condition. When denial ends, you may find that you are angry.

Anger

Anger is a normal emotional reaction to finding out that you have a chronic condition. It is natural to feel angry when you find out that there are no real explanations for why this has happened to you, what caused it, and the fact that there is no real cure. Uncertainty about the future and the potential threat to your independence and control may make you feel helpless, hopeless, and frustrated. It seems unfair, and you may ask yourself what you have done to deserve such a thing. You may find yourself lashing out at others for no apparent reason, leaving them confused and you frustrated.

Anger can be healthy if you release it in a healthy manner. Get it out in the open, express it non-aggressively to a friend, family member, health-care professional, or a support group who can listen and help you to "talk it through." Let those who are supporting you know that you are not angry at them, but at your arthritis. Trying to suppress anger can only increase stress levels and build resentment.

**Suppressing emotion seldom is successful—
find ways to release anger in a positive manner.**

If you can find a constructive way to spend the energy that is being fueled by anger, you are beating the arthritis. Find ways to release your anger; get in the shower and yell, pound a pillow (if it doesn't hurt your hands), go for a walk, exercise, write, paint, or find other new, creative outlets for your emotions.

Some anger may be caused by the threat that arthritis poses to the plans and expectations you had before your diagnosis. Having plans or expectations altered has undoubtedly happened to you throughout your life. Maybe you didn't make the baseball team so you took up swimming. Perhaps your employer's profits took an unexpected downward path, you were laid off, and subsequently you found another more satisfying job. It is likely that you have been in situations in the past that required you to change your plans, and it was not the end of the world. You survived those changes, and you will most likely survive the changes that an arthritis diagnosis imposes as well.

It can be very helpful if you focus on what you *can* still do and enjoy, not on what you *can't* do. The new activities that you find to replace the ones you can no longer do may be more interesting and enjoyable. One person was devastated that she could no longer downhill ski, but when she learned to cross-country ski on gentle terrain, using padded handles on her poles, she was delighted with the experience. She told her physical therapist that she had never realized the beauty of a trail beside a river, that taking it slower allowed her to enjoy nature, and that she felt more relaxed and satisfied after her outings than she used to feel after downhill sessions. This woman exchanged her original activity for one that better suited her current situation and, in doing so, let her anger go.

Bargaining

Bargaining sometimes comes at the same time as anger, or it may follow the anger stage. We all bargain differently. You may find yourself thinking, "I just can't give up bowling or tennis or my dance class. If I can keep doing those things, then I'll be grateful, and I'll never yell at my family again." You may make a bargain with a "higher power" to act a certain way if the higher power will prevent your arthritis from worsening—or better yet, cure you of the disease completely. This stage is usually short-lived, because you quickly come to realize that the bargaining is futile and your promises can't usually be kept. As you come to terms with your anger, you typically will dismiss bargaining as a viable option.

Depression

Everyone, healthy or not, feels a little sad or blue at times. A sad mood may be triggered by the weather, a distressing news story, or nothing in particular. The feeling passes somewhat like a thunder shower and life goes on. That is entirely normal. Typically, this form of depression lifts after a brief period. People with a systemic form of arthritis can also experience this kind of sadness as part of the disease process.

But there is another type of depression—called "reactive depression"—that is a response to a specific outside event. This sort of depression is triggered by events that affect your life in a negative way, such as a diagnosis of arthritis. Of course you are sad and upset when you get news like this! If you did *not* experience these feelings, there would be something wrong. You may experience fear, anxiety, frustration, and a sense of loss of control over your health and your life. Acknowledging that you are depressed is a healthy step toward gaining relief. Sometimes we don't recognize that we are depressed and try to adopt a cheerful front, hoping to cover what we are really feeling. We don't look for help, even if we need it, and we can begin to quietly and privately sink into despair.

**If you are depressed, make getting the help
you need to fight depression a number-one
priority in your health-management plan!**

How Do I Know If I Need Help?

You need to recognize depression before you can learn to manage
it. Ask yourself the following questions:

✦ Have I been feeling generally unhappy for more than six
weeks?

✦ Has my sleep pattern changed? Is my sleep interrupted? Am I
sleeping more than usual?

✦ Have my eating habits changed? Am I eating more than usual
or am I not interested in food? Am I losing/gaining weight?

✦ Am I withdrawing from social activities, hobbies, friends, and
fun?

✦ Do I feel listless and fatigued?

✦ Am I feeling worthless and/or guilty?

✦ Am I unable to concentrate and having difficulty making decisions?

✦ Am I neglecting my personal grooming?

✦ Am I experiencing problems regarding sexual activity?

✦ Do I think of death or even suicide?

If you have experienced some of these feelings in the past or
are currently experiencing them, you can be reassured that these

are very common feelings associated with a chronic illness and that help is available. These symptoms of depression can be dealt with, but first you must actively seek help.

You can put meaning and pleasure back into your life and deal with your emotions in a positive and lasting way. You—the person in control of your health—need to bring these feelings out in the open and talk about them to your health-care team, your doctor, your social worker, your support group, and even your friends and family. Communicate! It is difficult for your supporters to help if they have no idea what you are going through. You might not feel like it, but you need to initiate the process.

You are the person who is in control of your health-care plan! You must lead the parade to wellness.

What If I Am Depressed?

The following tips can help you fight your way out of the downward spiral of depression.

✦ Don't wallow in your depression, but do allow yourself to go through it. Give yourself time to feel the emotions, acknowledge them, and talk about them as honestly as possible.

✦ Acceptance will only come through understanding.

✦ Maintain an optimistic attitude, tough as it may be. Staying positive will lessen the stress that can relate to arthritis flare-ups.

✦ Don't look too far into the future—focus on what's happening now. If you are feeling sad, think of something that can make you laugh. Keep your sense of humor. Laughter really is a great medicine.

+ Continue with your daily routine. Get up, dress, do small chores, go out of the house or your apartment. Take a walk, pick up the mail, go shopping. Make plans, call a friend. Do these things even if you don't feel like it.

+ Engage in twenty to thirty minutes of physical activity each day.

+ Join a group—at church, in the community, in your neighborhood. Take a course, join a book club, or find a self-help group. Volunteer; studies show that people who are helping others are less depressed.

+ Plan a holiday, even if only for a day or two, to visit friends or relatives.

+ Do something nice for yourself every day. Watch a movie, read a book, do a crossword puzzle. Have a good cup of tea when you come back from a walk, and enjoy a favorite snack!

+ Get enough sleep. If you are having difficulty sleeping, make sure that your bed is comfortable; experiment with positions and pillows. Use your bedroom only for sleeping. If you can't sleep, leave the bedroom and sit in a comfortable chair to read or watch TV. Then go back to bed when you are more tired. Avoid using sleeping pills; they tend to lose effectiveness over time and can leave you with more sleep problems than you had to begin with. Avoid eating or drinking alcohol or caffeine around bedtime. Alcohol may help you to fall asleep initially, but it can actually disrupt your sleep later in the night. Instead of having a "night cap," develop a "before-bed routine." Take a warm bath, read a chapter, or practice relaxation techniques.

Signs of Serious Depression

It is great to take the steps outlined in the previous section to alleviate mild depression symptoms, but more severe symptoms require professional help. Certain behaviors or symptoms are indications that you need *urgent* assistance from a physician, a professional psychologist, a psychiatrist, a counselor, or a social worker. Substance abuse and suicidal thoughts are more extreme symptoms that call for extreme measures.

Excessive use of alcohol or pills is not healthy. Alcohol is a depressant; it may dull the ache temporarily, but it adds to the depression. If you are using alcohol to sleep or to manage pain, this is a warning sign. One or two drinks in the evening may help a person to relax and socialize, but if you need to drink alcohol throughout the day, you should get help. Talk to your doctor if you are abusing alcohol, or call Alcoholics Anonymous. If you are using narcotic painkillers or tranquilizers, be sure to discuss their safe use with your doctor or pharmacist. Many of these drugs have a depressant effect and only add to the problem. If you are taking antidepressants, be aware that in order to be effective, most must be used over a period of months or years, and sudden withdrawal from some of these drugs can be dangerous. Be sure to check with your doctor before you change or discontinue medications.

If you feel that you cannot go on, that you want to harm yourself or someone else, or that life is not worth living, **GET HELP!** Contact your health-care provider, a suicide hot line, a distress center, a friend, or a spiritual leader. Don't put it off! Sharing the burden or just talking about your feelings can lift an intolerable weight from your shoulders.

Acceptance

Once you have completed the journey through the stages of grief, you arrive at the blessing of acceptance. There is almost a sense of relief at coming to terms with your disease and knowing that you can move forward. You will have some bad days, but you will have many better days as well, and you may be surprised by the positive way in which your life changes once you accept your diagnosis.

Consider the example of Leo, a fifty-one-year-old man who had his own small painting and decorating business. Leo was forty-seven when rheumatoid arthritis hit him with a vengeance. Because of his need to support his family and his fears about his ability to do so in the long term, denial was his constant companion for a period of time. Finally, however, he could no longer ignore his disease. He was not able to climb ladders, reach to paint ceilings, or stoop to paint baseboards. He struggled on, hiring help to assist him, but found that when he took breaks to rest, so did his workers. His business began to lose money, and the stress resulted in frequent arthritis flare-ups. He was forced to give up the only work he had ever known. Leo was devastated, his self-esteem was in tatters, and the disease was wreaking havoc in his body. His rheumatologist and his physical therapist referred him to a vocational rehabilitation program. But he was denied access to the program because of his age! His wife called the social worker to say that she feared he was becoming suicidal.

The rheumatologist, social worker, and therapist persisted and appealed the decision, and Leo was finally accepted into a program to train microfilmers that guaranteed placement after training. He was so successful in his training that, at the end of the program, the agency added him to its staff and he became a trainer. His employer was supportive and understanding about the fact that he had to continue with his medical care and therapy and his occasional need for time off. After a few years, Leo visited his physical therapist at her office to tell her about how much he enjoyed his new career, how much happier he was, and how well he and his family were doing. He said, "What I thought was the worst possible affliction for me has turned out to be a blessing in disguise. Of course, I would prefer not to have arthritis, but if I didn't have it, I wouldn't have had the opportunity to do such satisfying work and enjoy a job so much." Leo is a man who moved through the stages of grief and was finally able to enjoy acceptance.

**Sometimes, what appears to be a disaster
is a blessing in disguise.**

WHAT SHOULD I DO ABOUT ALL THESE FEELINGS?

Be open. Talk openly about the feelings you have surrounding your condition. Your personal support system, friends, family, and health-care team are there to help you over the hurdles.

Learn all you can about your disease and its management. Knowledge about your condition is the most powerful tool you can use to fight the effects of arthritis. Knowledge will give you the power and strength to move through these feelings and come to grips with the future.

Take responsibility for your role in your emotional state. Each person's personal psychology influences to a great degree how well or how ill he or she feels. Many people with severe disabling disorders report that they are somewhat satisfied or very satisfied with their lives. At the same time, there are many who, while not seriously ill, consider themselves disabled and are dissatisfied with their health. This disparity can be explained partially by our psychological makeup and our beliefs, expectations, and experiences, as well as the culture in which we were raised. If, as a child, you were rushed to the doctor for every sniffle or stomachache, you may become an adult who is more likely to see minor symptoms as significant and severe than a person who has been raised in an environment where the expectations are that no one will escape the usual aches, pains, and illnesses of life.

Your own attitude toward your illness may determine how fulfilling your life can be with arthritis.

Be positive. Your own coping mechanisms—that is, how you deal with stress, uncertainty, or disappointment—will affect how you adjust to your diagnosis. If you have always had an optimistic, positive outlook, you will likely cope better than if you have a tendency to look on the dark side of life's situations. Try to be a person who deals with situations in a positive way, and you just may find things working out better than you had thought they could.

Be realistic. Unrealistic expectations about health and medical care can lead to disappointment when we compare them with real life. By understanding the social pressures and the unrealistic expectations created by a profit-oriented, marketing society, you take the first steps toward coping better with your symptoms. In the United States and Canada, there have been extraordinary medical advances in the past decades. We also live in a culture where we are constantly bombarded with information about drugs that claim to be able to turn your life around, and to keep you young, healthy, and attractive forever. As a result, many North Americans have expectations that we all will be cured of every ill and dance into a retirement community to play tennis and golf and live in comfort, seemingly forever. The reality is that daily life often contains its fair share of allergies, insomnia, aches, and pains. Many conditions cannot be "fixed."

Our tendency is to compare ourselves upward, with the TV images of the perfect body and a vigorous and active life. While high expectations for activity can lead us to more exciting lifestyle pursuits than our parents and grandparents enjoyed, they can also make us intolerant or unrealistic about the limitations our bodies can impose on us. Gracefully accepting those limitations and learning to live a fulfilling life within realistic parameters is the ultimate goal for people who have arthritis. Your health does not belong to TV commercials, sensational media reports, pharmaceutical advertising, or even to your health-care providers. **Your health belongs to you!** You can take control, and you can ask for help.

Looking Forward

This chapter has explained the effects that arthritis can have on your emotional health and well-being and has offered suggestions to help you and others deal with those effects. The next chapter addresses even more sensitive aspects of your life—your intimate relationships. Chapter 15 offers reassurance and practical advice to help you manage this important area of your life and will be valuable to you as you deal with the physical changes that may challenge your relationships.

Chapter 15

Enjoying Happy and Healthy Intimate Relationships

A chronic disease such as arthritis, which involves pain and fatigue and limits your mobility, can negatively affect self-esteem and self-image. It also may cause anxiety and depression. These are decidedly unromantic feelings that can sabotage your sexuality and deprive you of the pleasures and comforts of love-making. Your intimate relationships may undergo changes if pain and depression cause you to withdraw from social activities or physical challenges, especially if physical limitations or changes make you shy or self-conscious around others. It can be difficult and frustrating to try to explain your condition to the people around you—especially so if you are dating and trying to establish new relationships. Even established intimate relationships may stumble in the face of an arthritis diagnosis.

Forty percent of people with rheumatoid arthritis say that this condition causes difficulty in their love-making. But it is not OK to let intimate relations fall by the wayside. The formation and

327

maintenance of healthy relationships is an important aspect of disease management. Loving partners can help you beat depression, distract you from pain, and support you when you need love. Research has shown that the people with arthritis who do best are those who have strong support systems. Studies also indicate that having good emotional support actually improves your physical health.

This chapter is aimed at helping you address not only the physical challenges of intimacy, but also the emotions that you and your partner may experience as this uninvited guest—arthritis—attempts to invade your relationship. It also provides suggestions for things that you and your partner can do together to grow and strengthen your relationship in spite of the intrusion of a chronic illness.

WHERE DO WE START?

In our society, it is not always easy to bring up personal topics. At the same time, we know that it is difficult, if not impossible, to address sensitive issues if they are not discussed openly and directly. In this chapter, we attempt to be frank and honest and, at the same time, make our discussion of these sensitive issues as discomfort-free as possible. The following information can help you get started in addressing the important issue of arthritis and intimacy if it is something that is affecting your life.

Studies show that issues relating to sexual intimacy are relevant for many people with arthritis. The disease itself seldom causes loss of desire, but the physical effects and the emotional stress can seriously affect sexual needs, ability, and satisfaction for both partners. Figure 15.1 illustrates the cascade of reactions that can occur as a result of arthritis affecting your sexuality. In the figure, you can see how low self-esteem, avoidance of intimacy, and depression can feed on each other and result in a vicious cycle of negative emotions and behaviors.

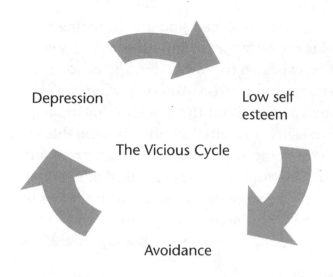

Figure 15.1
Emotions have a way of building up and feeding on each other so that it becomes difficult to break the vicious cycle and find relief.

Depression

Low self esteem

The Vicious Cycle

Avoidance

Talk About It!

If you have experienced changes in your desire for intimacy or your response to the advances of your partner since you learned about your arthritis, these may be due to a number of factors, both physical and emotional. Sometimes it is easier for the person with arthritis and his or her partner to try to ignore the symptoms or hope that they will just disappear. An important first step is to accept the reality of the situation. Partners need to acknowledge that there is a problem and talk about it. The first step to solving an intimacy issue is to *communicate.* You can't fix what you don't acknowledge. If you don't communicate, or if you deny the problem, it will get worse, not better.

If you are the person with the disease, you need to know how your partner is feeling. Your partner may be reluctant to initiate sexual activity because of fear of causing increased pain, or because he or she is too caught up in the stages of grieving described in Chapter 14. It is important to understand that, although your partner may go through these stages just like you, he or she may not be in the same stage at the same time that you are. Initiating conversation about intimacy is not always easy, but it needs to happen.

Your partner cannot be expected to read your mind or to anticipate your needs, so you need to be direct. You may want to begin by telling him or her how you feel about the changes that are happening to you both physically and emotionally. You might say something like: "There are some days when the pain from my arthritis just makes doing the simplest things very difficult. Asking for help makes me feel badly, so sometimes I just wait until I'm so frustrated that I get angry and blow up. I'm not angry at you—I am angry at the disease."

Acknowledge and share your feelings.

Listen to what your partner says, verbalize your own feelings and reactions, and give feedback on his or her comments. Responding in this way lets your partner know that he or she has been heard and acknowledged. You are in this together, and you need to talk about it!

Learn About It!

Once you have openly discussed your reactions to the arthritis, the next step is to educate yourself and your partner so that you can become knowledgeable about the effects of arthritis, both physical and emotional. Your partner needs to know about the treatments that you are receiving, their potential effects, and how long it may take for them to be effective. You may feel that you don't want to burden those close to you with all of the details, but if you don't share this information, they will be less equipped to support you. Lack of knowledge about the illness, its effects, and its treatment may prevent a partner from being supportive of a person who has arthritis. Research into couples who are dealing with chronic illness shows that those who adjust the best are those who are educated about the disease and its treatment and are supportive of each other.

If you are not comfortable talking about your arthritis and treatment, you can provide your partner and/or friends with educational materials that are available from your doctor, your healthcare provider, or The Arthritis Foundation and The Arthritis Society. Both organizations have excellent web sites with downloadable information on almost everything you could want to know, including brochures and information on sexuality.

Attending an arthritis self-management program together can help you and your partner understand arthritis and its treatment. It can help open your lines of communication as you discover that the other participants experience similar challenges. Other participants can also offer recommendations and solutions. One researcher observed that the people who benefited the most from self-help groups were those who attended with their partner.

How Do I Talk to My Physician About Intimacy?

If lack of desire, fear, pain, or depression is getting in the way of intimacy, this is the time to get the answers from someone knowledgeable about sexuality and arthritis. The most obvious place to go for information might be your rheumatologist or primary-care physician.

You need to find out from your physician if sexual issues are due to the effects of the disease, your feelings about the disease, or the medications you are taking. Even doctors are not always comfortable discussing sexuality, so you may need to initiate the process. At the very least, a physician should acknowledge your concerns and provide information that will help answer your questions. If health-care professionals do not respond in a way that is helpful to you, remember that you have the right to ask for a referral to someone who can help.

Your doctor is there to help or to refer you to someone who can. The more open you can be, the more help you can expect to receive.

Ideally, both partners should go to the appointment and be prepared to openly discuss topics such as:

✦ Changes in sexual desire or response.

✦ Feelings of depression and lack of interest in sexual activity.

✦ Concerns partners may have about experiencing or causing pain during intimacy.

✦ How fatigue may be affecting desire.

✦ Medication usage and potential side effects.

A Word About Sexuality and Medications

Your physician or pharmacist will be able to inform you about the possible effects your medication may be having on your sexual desires and abilities.

There are two issues to consider in this regard:

✦ Pain medication needs to be taken so that medication is at its most effective when you wish to be intimate. At the same time, you want to make sure that pain medication is not inhibiting desire by dulling your senses.

✦ Some medications—such as antidepressants, corticosteroids, muscle relaxants, and others—can inhibit your sex drive and the ability to achieve an orgasm, have and maintain an erection, or ejaculate.

Some medications can inhibit sex drive.

Review the effects that your medications may have on your sex drive with your physician. You don't need to choose between effective medication and satisfactory sexual relations. The answer may be an adjustment of the dosage, the timing of the doses, or a change to a different drug.

Can Other Health-Care Professionals Help Me?

Other people who can help you deal with sexuality and intimacy issues include the following:

✦ Social workers can help couples come to terms with the emotional aspects of chronic diseases and the adjustments necessary to life roles and relationships.

✦ Physical therapists and nurses, particularly those experienced in arthritis, can suggest relaxation techniques and pain-management strategies to help people to prepare for love-making. They can also work with you to find positions for intercourse that can be satisfying without causing pain or putting extra stress on joints.

✦ Psychologists can be of great assistance in dealing with depression—one of the most common causes of lack of sexual desire and satisfaction. They also offer marriage or couple-counseling services to support partners in building a healthy relationship outside of the bedroom.

Caution is advised in choosing counseling services. In many states and provinces, unqualified persons may advertise psychosocial therapy or counseling that may be of limited usefulness, serving only to line the pockets of the individuals who provide bogus services. Be sure to check the credentials of any person providing health-care or counseling services.

FACING FEARS

Fear of the unknown can cause partners to avoid really considering, and therefore dealing with, the effects of arthritis on the sexual aspects of their relationship. Worried about how this chronic illness is going to change their lives, they may try to ignore it. Directly addressing concerns and learning about arthritis and its effects can bring a couple to a new understanding of sexuality. Strange as it may seem, facing this problem and looking for solutions together can actually improve your sex life. As you explore your sensuality and try out new ways to stimulate each other both emotionally and physically, you may ultimately discover that your relationship becomes more satisfying.

A willingness to accept the limitations of the person with the disease is extremely helpful and gets things out into the open. Couples who can realistically deal with the facts can begin to develop the mutual coping skills to deal effectively with fears.

What About the Pain?

Not surprisingly, the most common fear about sexual intimacy for people with arthritis is the pain that they may experience during love-making. Pain can be distressing and mood-altering. You may think that, if simply holding hands is painful, how can I conceive of enjoying sexual contact? In this case, avoidance becomes an understandable reaction. A fear of causing pain can be worrisome to the partner without arthritis. As a result, he or she may cease initiating intimacy and may begin to harbor resentment. Both partners can end up feeling miserable, resentful, and guilty for denying the other one of life's most pleasurable experiences. Talking to each other in a caring manner, with sensitivity about the fears that both partners are facing, is essential. Just as turning on the light and checking out that frightening shadow in the corner is better than pretending it's not there, turning on the light and exposing your lurking fears about intimacy can be a very good thing.

Am I Still Attractive?

Very often, the partner with arthritis experiences a real blow to his or her self-image and sense of self-worth. He or she may feel less physically attractive as a result of changes to the joints or due to the side effects of medication. He or she may no longer feel like a whole, functioning person. This can lead a person to avoid intimacy, due to the fear that his or her partner may not find the person attractive or that he or she may not be able to perform adequately.

If you are fighting this fear, you are not alone. Studies have shown that most women, healthy or not, are embarrassed by some part of their body. Men often experience these feelings as well. Do not guess at what your partner's feelings are. Your partner, who found you attractive in the first place, likely sees beyond the physical changes. Both partners need to talk openly about these concerns so that they can relieve fears and move forward. In a mature relationship, sexual attraction is based on more than physical appearances.

**Real intimacy is based on more
than physical appearances.**

To improve your self-image and beat down those negative feelings, find ways that allow you to feel good *inside* your body. Do things that make you feel good about yourself. Have a warm bubble bath, have your hair done, wear clothes that are comfortable and attractive, light candles, or read a romantic poem or story. Get some exercise and trigger some of those "feel-good" hormones. The better you feel in your body, the more you will enjoy your sexuality.

Can I Still Perform?

Men with arthritis, while they typically may worry less about body image, often have fears about their ability to perform sexually. Discussing these fears with your partner is important and helpful. Pain, depression, or medication may interfere with the ability to have or maintain an erection. This situation should be discussed with your physician, particularly if the culprit is your medication. A change in medication or in the timing of the dosage may solve the problem. Both partners should also be aware that while an erection is necessary for intercourse, an orgasm is achievable without an erection. And, of course, intimacy does not necessarily require intercourse.

Intimacy does not require intercourse.

For women, some forms of medication can cause decreased vaginal lubrication, causing pain on penetration. The use of a sterile lubricating jelly can alleviate this difficulty.

Will I Be Left Alone?

Experts say that chronically ill men and women have fears that their partner will abandon them because of their physical limitations. These fears lead to the greater fear that they may end up on their own, with no one caring for them. Chronically ill people may become concerned that their partners will leave them for healthier people who can do more physically.

These fears need to be addressed in a very sensitive and caring way. You need to tell your partner that you are worried and ask for reassurance. In most cases, the response will relieve your fears. However, if you do not get reassurance, it is better to know where you stand so that you can make choices accordingly and seek support elsewhere. While chronic illness can be hard on a partnership, it is typically not enough to turn a solid relationship into a bad one. A partner who is unfaithful once you have been diagnosed with a chronic disease might very well have been unfaithful whether or not you became ill. In this situation, you may need to find a qualified counselor to help you and your partner over these hurdles, addressing all your relationship concerns, not just those that have been accentuated by your illness.

Once you have dealt with your fears, you will feel much more confident and ready to move on with your intimate relationship.

ARTHRITIS AND PREGNANCY

For people of child-bearing age, thinking about the future naturally includes concerns about family planning and the potential implications of the disease in terms of conception, pregnancy, and childbirth. Couples who want to begin a family should consult a physician about their plans. In particular, they should ask about any medications they currently take and whether these need to be discontinued or changed.

In most cases, pregnancy does not result in a worsening of arthritis. In fact, women with rheumatoid arthritis often feel better during pregnancy; some are even able to stop their medications during gestation. In the late stages of pregnancy, the back and leg joints may be uncomfortable due to the extra weight putting stress on these joints. This can usually be managed with extra rest and maintenance of good posture. Women with arthritis rarely require a cesarean section due to joint damage and usually can expect to have an uncomplicated delivery.

For some women, symptoms of arthritis are lessened during pregnancy.

It is not uncommon for women to experience a flare-up of their arthritis following delivery. Do not despair if this happens, as the flare-up usually subsides. It may be wise to prepare for this eventuality by organizing some extra help during this period. A consultation with an occupational therapist might also be helpful, as he or she can provide pointers on caring for a baby while you also protect your joints and conserve your energy. Arthritis does not have negative effects on the baby's *in utero* development except possibly in the case of a mother with lupus. Women with lupus can have children but need to be closely monitored by a rheumatologist and an obstetrician. If you have lupus and are considering starting a family, consult your physician before becoming pregnant.

AM I READY FOR INTIMACY?

You can't begin to find pleasure in your sexuality if you fear being hurt. Therefore, it is vital that both partners share an understanding of what feels good to each person and what causes pain. Once you are comfortable talking with your partner about how each of you feels about arthritis and your sexuality, you will be ready to find solutions.

Take the Time to Reawaken Romance

One expert in the field of sexuality suggests that the best way to revive the romance in your life is to sit with your partner, with your clothes on, and talk about the things that each of you does to make the other feel loved and cared for. Talk also about the things that you would like the other to begin to do—things that you will find reassuring and comforting in the face of the difficulties created by arthritis.

Reminisce. Talking about times in your lives that have created happy memories and the feelings that these memories evoke can help you to focus on the positives and rekindle the flame. Share a glass of wine, play some soft music, and turn the lights low.

Don't rush to the bedroom! Simply relaxing together on the couch, in a position in which the person with arthritis is comfortable, can pave the way to intimacy. Be patient, take your time, and share your thoughts and feelings. Just holding hands gently or stroking an arm, a cheek, or a shoulder can be a reassuring and healing experience. Sensuality engages the mind as much as the body; when the mind is ready, the body will respond more willingly.

Make sure that both your mind and your body are ready for intimacy.

If you are the parents of young children (or even not-so-young children) or have an extended family with whom you live, you may benefit from a weekend getaway or a longer holiday. A relaxing setting with a minimum of distractions or interruptions can be a wonderful tonic and provide an opportunity to rekindle romantic feelings.

To the Bedroom

Talking together about what kinds of physical stimulation you enjoy, which positions you find most comfortable, and even what fantasies you find most arousing can be a wonderful distraction from pain and stiffness and is a bonding experience for both partners. Move toward the bedroom only when you are relaxed and ready. The room should be warm. You may need plenty of pillows to support your body so that it is relaxed and comfortable. Be patient, don't rush, and don't expect things to go perfectly. It will take some experimentation, and that can be fun!

The unrealistic portrayal manufactured by the media of love-making as an exhausting, athletic marathon is just that—unrealistic. In addition to being physically satisfying, sex can be gentle, tender, and healing. Romantic times and intimacy can be even more satisfying than intercourse itself.

Your skin is the largest sensual organ in the body, with millions of sensory nerve endings. Touch on almost any place on the body can be very arousing and comforting. Having a partner massage you gently, perhaps with scented oil when you are tired and aching, can be very romantic. If you remind yourself that sexuality is as much in the mind as in the body, you can be creative and tender in your approach as you explore each other's body with touch and discover what each finds desirable.

Sexual stimulation and touching can occur in almost any position and can be heightened by the use of lotions, oils, feathers, fur, or various sex "toys." The lips, earlobes, neck, breasts, and insides of arms or thighs are particularly erogenous (i.e., sensitive to sexual stimulation) areas. Some prefer light touch, while others enjoy a firmer touch. Many people are aroused by the touch of the lips, the tongue, or a sex toy. You are limited only by your imagination and by what is acceptable to you as a couple.

Controlling Symptoms

Nobody wants their sexual pleasure to be interrupted by arthritis symptoms. This means that romantic encounters may require some advance planning. This obviously takes the spontaneity out of the situation, but you can think of the planning as getting ready for a date! Plan your love-making for the time of day that you generally feel best, and avoid extra activities that could leave you fatigued. Try some gentle range-of-motion and stretching exercises to relieve stiffness, or take a warm shower.

Planning ahead can help things go more smoothly.

There may still be times when love-making can be spontaneous, such as when you are having a good day and are feeling better. If this occurs, make the most of it.

To control pain, time your medications to be at their most effective when you are anticipating sexual activity. Some medications—such as narcotic drugs, muscle relaxants, and tranquilizers—may dull your senses. You really don't want this to happen if you plan on being intimate. An alternative way to block out pain is to use fantasy to distract you from pain. If you can focus on the erotic and emotional sensations, the pain is no longer able to distract you. You may choose to get some guidance from an expert in visualization techniques to get you started.

Use fantasy to distract yourself from the pain.

To keep symptoms from interfering with sexual activities, you need to find positions that are comfortable for both partners. These are best found through experimentation. Many of the problems that come from joint pain are caused by mechanical problems, and these can be solved by using adapted or new positions for intercourse. Common problems usually involve painful or restricted movement in the lower back and hips. Figures 15.2 and 15.3 provide examples of positions that may be acceptable to people with low-back or lower-limb arthritis, especially in the hips. There are several well-illustrated books available in bookstores that can also help you find different positions that may work for you.

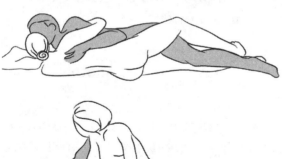

Figure 15.2a
The couple is side-by-side,
with front entry.

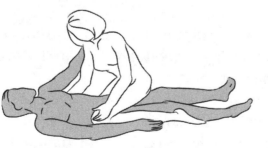

Figure 15.2b
The man is on his back; the
woman is on top, supporting
her own weight, either facing
him or with her back to him.
This position is good if the man
is unable to support his weight
with his upper limbs.

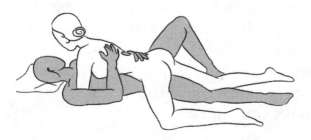

Figure 15.2c
This position works if
the man has problems
on one side only.

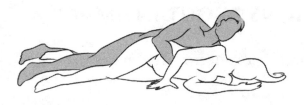

Figure 15.3a
The couple is side-by-side
with rear entry.

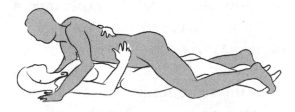

Figure 15.3b
This position works if the
woman is unable to move her
legs apart. Here the man
supports his own weight, with
front entry.

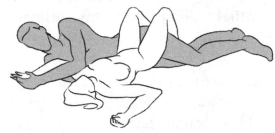

Figure 15.3c
This position, with rear entry,
may work for women with
severe hip and knee
contractures.

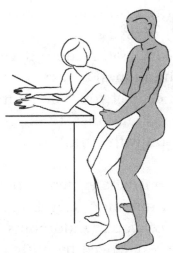

Figure 15.3d
This is a standing position.
The couple is supported by
furniture, with rear entry.

Figure 15.3e
This position involves kneeling,
with rear entry, and should
be avoided if there is pain in the
upper limbs for the front partner.

OTHER QUESTIONS ABOUT INTIMACY

The following list addresses other concerns that may create barriers to sexual intimacy.

+ **What if intercourse is not possible?** If, despite experimentation with positioning, it is not possible to have intercourse, there are other means of achieving orgasm. Manual or oral stimulation, focusing on a variety of erogenous zones of the body, can often bring about the same result. Remember that any techniques that you as a couple find comfortable, pleasurable, and satisfying are entirely acceptable; the intimacy belongs to you and no one else.

+ **What about orgasm?** Contrary to the popular myth that sexual intimacy, to be successful, must include simultaneous orgasm for both partners, some individuals report that they enjoy closeness and intimacy as much as, or more than, orgasm. However, it is worth being creative in your pursuit of orgasm if you have arthritis. An orgasm, while not essential to satisfaction, does cause a surge of endorphins (feel good hormones) that evoke a feeling of well-being and can alleviate or distract you from joint pain. This effect can last from forty-five minutes to three hours—a pleasant side effect for the person with arthritis.

+ **What if there is no partner?** In situations where there is no sexual partner, self-stimulation or masturbation can bring about orgasm and the release of those "feel-good" endorphins. According to statistics, self-stimulation is practiced by a high percentage of individuals in order to meet sexual needs. For arthritis patients, as well as the general public, there are no harmful consequences from masturbation.

✦ **What about surgery?** Arthritis in the hip can be a painful barrier to intercourse. Undergoing a hip replacement can bring significant relief. Most people can resume sexual activities six weeks after hip-replacement surgery but need to continue to avoid certain positions. If you have surgery, your surgeon or therapist will most likely have provided you with instructions about positioning. If not, be sure to ask.

✦ **What about abstinence?** The decision to abstain from sexual activity because of your chronic pain or because sex is not of interest to you is a choice that some people make. It is, however, important to your relationship with your partner and needs to be a shared decision. This is a situation requiring good communication with mutual support and understanding. You may find it helpful to seek some counseling from a qualified person who has skills in dealing with interpersonal relationships.

Having arthritis can require you and your partner to make adjustments to many aspects of your lives, including your sexual relationship. It takes courage to get the issues out in the open. However, when you openly discuss your problems and needs with mutual thoughtfulness, and when you work through them together, you can come to a new understanding of intimacy and explore new possibilities for building your relationship. Be patient with each other and enjoy the experience as you experiment with positioning and new techniques. Remember that where there is a will, there is a way. Work on the will first; the way will naturally follow. For many couples, the process of rediscovery necessitated by a diagnosis of arthritis has resulted in a more satisfying and meaningful intimate relationship.

Looking Forward

This chapter has provided information to help you maintain your intimate relationship in the face of an arthritis diagnosis. Healthy relationships are an important part of wellness. Chapter 16 will provide you with more information on other important aspects of wellness and will give you useful suggestions for how you can live a healthy and fulfilling life with arthritis.

Chapter 16

Making Healthy Lifestyle Choices

The World Health Organization defines health promotion as "enabling people to increase control over and to improve their health." In the United States and Canada, governments at all levels, recognizing that the burden of chronic disease is rapidly growing, are actively promoting health and healthy lifestyles as strategies to prevent disease and disability. The Bill of Rights for People with Arthritis outlined in Chapter 4 states that people with arthritis have the *responsibility to pursue healthy lifestyles*. In the spirit of health promotion, this chapter is intended to help you as the leader of your health-care team make the healthy choices that can help prevent or delay disability and improve your overall health.

Throughout this book, we have written extensively about the physical and emotional changes that can take place in your life when you have arthritis. Whether you are diagnosed with a mild form of osteoarthritis, a painful case of fibromyalgia, or severe inflammatory arthritis, you will probably need to make some changes in your exercise habits, your work life, your diet, and your recreational and social activities. An arthritis diagnosis is a good reason to take a closer look at your lifestyle and think about ways in which you can make healthy changes. Doing so helps ensure that you can be in "good shape for the shape you're in."

KEY LIFESTYLE ISSUES

While you may not be in control of many of the changes that take place in your body and in your abilities as a result of arthritis, you *are* in control of your lifestyle. You can decide to make healthy choices that will make a difference in how you manage your life with arthritis.

Take a closer look at your lifestyle to ensure that you are in good shape for the shape you are in.

Before you can make healthy changes in your lifestyle, you may need to take an inventory of the habits and activities in your life that could benefit from some improvement. How you choose to manage the following key lifestyle issues can make a measurable difference in your quality of life:

+ **Diet.** Maintaining a healthy weight can be difficult. It is something with which many people struggle—even those without arthritis. In the early stages of inflammatory arthritis, the systemic nature of the illness may decrease your appetite, or you may just not feel like preparing meals; in this case, weight loss may occur as a result of poor nutrition. On the other hand, some arthritis patients gain weight because inactivity and weight gain often go hand in hand. As you become less active, you burn fewer calories. As you gain weight, you may become even less active. This is a vicious cycle, and you should do your best to break it. Being overweight puts you at risk for numerous illnesses (like diabetes and high blood pressure) and puts added strain on your already taxed joints.

✦ **Exercise habits.** Pain, stiffness, depression, and an inability to participate in physical activities that you previously enjoyed may make you less inclined to exercise. This can result in a loss of strength, mobility, and energy. Inactivity perpetuates itself and can lead to more health problems, such as weight gain, depression, disability, osteoporosis, high blood pressure, and diabetes. Regular physical activity considerably lowers your risk of developing these conditions.

✦ **Stress management.** Many things can cause stress, such as a job change, moving, or the death of a loved one. Most people think about stress mainly in terms of these negative events in their lives, but there are also positive sources of stress, such as weddings, childbirth, and job promotions. Stress is a normal part of life. It is the reaction of your mind and body to problems, changes, and other pressures. While stress is a normal part of life, too much stress due to negative events can cause you to experience more pain and make dealing with the challenges of a chronic disease like arthritis all the more difficult. If you have arthritis, you have an additional stress that people without a chronic disease do not face. By learning to recognize and manage stress in a positive way, you can reduce pain and feel healthier.

Manage your stress in a positive way:
Strive for "stress without distress."

✦ **Balance.** A balance between work and play, and activity and rest, is essential to a healthy lifestyle. Studies have shown that workers who maintain a balance between their work life and their time off are more efficient, productive, and generally healthier than those who do not take breaks or vacations. It is important for people with arthritis to recognize that rest is a positive thing when it is balanced with appropriate exercise and activity.

✦ **Alcohol and medication abuse and tobacco use.** The moderate enjoyment of alcohol is not problematic unless you have been advised not to drink alcohol while taking certain medications, such as methotrexate. Pain relievers, tranquilizers, and antidepressants must always be taken as prescribed. We all know of the risks that smoking imposes on the cardiovascular system and the respiratory system, but many do not know that smoking has been shown to have an increased negative effect on people with rheumatoid arthritis. Banishing unhealthy habits can have a very immediate and positive effect on your wellness.

SETTING *SMART* GOALS

Make a list of the aspects surrounding your lifestyle that you want and need to change. Once you have identified these things, you can begin to make a contract with yourself about how you will make changes. Setting goals is a strong beginning. These goals should be SMART: specific, measurable, attainable, relevant, and time-oriented.

An example of a SMART goal is shown in Table 16.1. Notice that each element of the SMART goal is reasonable. By starting with reasonable expectations, you avoid setting yourself up for disappointment, and each time you achieve a goal, you can reward yourself and set a new one.

Table 16.1
Example of a SMART Goal

Specific	I will lose weight.
Measurable	I will lose five pounds.
Attainable	This much weight loss is possible.
Relevant	Weight loss will reduce my risk of other illness and may reduce pain.
Time-oriented	I can do this in one month.

Looking at the key elements of lifestyle and understanding their importance in relation to living with arthritis will help you get started and reach your goals.

MAKING GOOD CHOICES ABOUT DIET AND NUTRITION

You may have heard numerous claims that certain special diets, types of foods, or dietary supplements can aggravate or cure arthritis. Some of these claims are fraudulent; others have not been adequately tested. Some diets that claim to heal arthritis can even have harmful effects because they eliminate certain nutrients that are essential to good health. Be skeptical of any diet that claims to be a cure for arthritis or that suggests that you eliminate any complete food groups (such as fats or carbohydrates or proteins). See Chapter 18 for more information on avoiding unproven cures.

**Be skeptical of any diet that
claims to cure your arthritis.**

Regardless of the unanswered questions relating to certain types of diets, there is no doubt that all people with arthritis can benefit from eating a healthy, well-balanced diet. Both the American and the Canadian governments provide excellent guides for healthy eating and activity. MyPyramid in the United States (www.mypyramid.gov) and The Guide to Healthy Eating and Physical Activity in Canada (www.eatwellbeactive.gc.ca) are readily available at no cost from the respective web sites. They are also available in libraries, at doctors' offices, and in many public-health facilities. These guides offer numerous healthy eating tips and describe the amount of food you need every day, depending on how physically active you are as well as your body size, your age, and your gender. Following these guides is easy, as they contain information on how to gauge portion sizes and understand nutrition labels, which are now required for foods in both countries.

What Foods Are Part of a Healthy Diet?

Enjoy a variety of healthy foods from the food groups in Table 16.2.

If you are inactive, pay attention to portion sizes as well as to the number of portions rather than eliminating foods from any of the food groups. All people, active or inactive, require good nutrition. The following list can help you choose appropriate portion sizes.

✦ One cup of fruit is equal to the size of your fist.

✦ Three ounces of meat is the size of a deck of cards and can fit onto the palm of your hand.

Table 16.2
Recommended Servings for Food Groups

FOOD GROUP	RECOMMENDED AMOUNTS FOR A PERSON WHO IS CONSUMING 2,000 CALORIES PER DAY
Whole-grain products: bread, grains, or pasta.	Six to nine one-ounce servings of whole-grain products per day. In general, at least half of the grains should come from whole grains.
Vegetables and fruit: dark green, red, or orange.	Two cups of fruit and two cups of vegetables per day. Choose a variety of fruits and vegetables each day. In particular, select from all five vegetable subgroups (dark green, orange, legumes, starchy vegetables, and other vegetables) several times a week.
Milk products: low-fat cheese, milk, or yogurt.	Three cups per day of fat-free or low-fat milk or equivalent milk products.
Protein sources: fish, poultry, meat, peanut butter, legumes, or tofu.	Five and one-half to six ounces of protein per day.

MEASURE YOUR PORTIONS TO MAKE SURE THAT YOU
ARE STAYING WITHIN THE GUIDELINES.

✦ One ounce of meat or cheese is the size of a pair of dice.

✦ One ounce of nuts can be held in your cupped hand. A half cup of rice or pasta is the size of an ice-cream scoop or half of a tennis ball.

What Foods Should I Enjoy Only in Moderation?

Some foods and beverages are not part of the four food groups and should be enjoyed only in moderation because they are high in fat or sugars. Fatty and sweet foods are high in calories but relatively low in the nutrients and fiber that your body needs to function well. Fat and sugar disproportionately contribute to the number of calories that people consume. Foods such as jam, honey, candies, soft drinks, and fruit-flavored drinks have a high sugar content. Butter, margarine, and some cooking oils are high in fat content. Many snack foods and baked goods are prepared with these and/or with excess salt and should be eaten only in moderation. Snack foods are also highly processed and contain refined white flours and trans fats, both of which are high in calories but low in nutritional value. These foods fill you up less than whole grains and good fats (like olive oil) and yet are full of calories. Avoid processed foods, and try to "eat fresh" whenever you can. As a general rule of thumb, the less processing a food product has been through, the more nutritious (and delicious) it will be.

Eat fresh!

What About Weight-Loss Diets?

Almost everywhere you look, advertisements in television, newspapers, and magazines are promoting new "magical" weight-loss schemes. Some weight-loss programs promise the loss of 70 to 100 pounds in a very short time, and products from electrical stimulators to pills promise to melt the pounds away. The truth is that losing weight and maintaining a healthy weight is accomplished by limiting calories, eating a balanced diet, and regularly engaging in moderate exercise. If you are concerned about being overweight or obese, this recipe for a healthy lifestyle is the only path proven to produce longer-lasting benefits. And implementing this plan costs far less than fad diets or devices as well!

If a diet promises a result that seems to be too good to be true, it probably is.

If you have a chronic condition such as arthritis, or any other health condition, solicit the advice of a professional health-care provider before you undertake a weight-loss program. People come in all shapes, sizes, and weights, and a weight-loss plan that is good for one person is not necessarily good for another. Talk to your doctor about what weight is right for you, and discuss any plans for changing how you eat or exercise so that you can make a realistic plan to achieve a weight-loss goal. A dietitian or nutritionist can analyze your current caloric intake and, based on your body build, general health, and age, help you get on track.

Modifying your lifestyle to make healthy choices and lose weight can be one of the most difficult challenges you will face. It may mean giving up old habits like daily snacking on potato chips, having donuts with your coffee every morning, and overindulging in other foods that are low in nutritional value but high in satisfaction and calories. A glass of water is usually less tempting than a soft drink, but the dividends are enormous when you make a healthy choice.

**Eating right and exercising are easier if you
find a friend and use the "buddy system."**

Start slowly. Gradual, consistent weight loss will help your body to adjust and, in the long run, will help you to stay positive and to keep at it. Once you have achieved your weight-loss goal, you will find it easier to maintain a healthy weight. Celebrate success along the way, and keep a realistic perspective. Maintain an active and varied lifestyle while working toward your weight-loss and exercise goals. Becoming obsessed with weight and neglecting other aspects of life is stressful and unhealthy.

Seek out support from family and friends. You may even find a friend who wants to join you on this journey to a healthy lifestyle. Having a weight-loss "buddy" is a proven strategy for success. You can encourage and support each other.

How Can I Maintain a Healthy Weight?

When you have reached your weight-loss goal, it is important to develop a plan for keeping off the weight. The following tips can help you maintain a healthy weight.

✦ Maintain a reasonable caloric intake after you have met your weight-loss goal. Do not go back to your pre-diet portion sizes or food choices. Reduced fat and calorie intake is critical.

✦ Keep track of your food intake. It is easy to slip back if you are unaware of what you are eating. Most successful "losers" resort to a food log or diary when they are concerned that their weight may be creeping back up. Writing down what you eat, when you eat it, keeps you aware of what you are eating and can help you to keep mindless snacking under control.

✦ Stay physically active. Engage in an exercise regime that you enjoy. Change your exercise habits if you get bored. Try new activities, take classes, and get outdoors in nice weather.

✦ Eat breakfast every day. Research has shown that people who eat breakfast do better at keeping off the weight.

DEVELOPING GOOD EXERCISE HABITS

The importance of exercise as a cornerstone in the management of arthritis has been emphasized in several chapters of this book already, but we truly believe that it is difficult to overemphasize its importance. Physical activity and healthy eating are recognized as the cornerstones to a healthy lifestyle for people who have arthritis.

The immediate benefits of beginning regular physical activity include:

✦ Meeting other people.

✦ Feeling more relaxed.

✦ Sleeping better.

✦ Having fun.

A continued commitment to regular physical activity provides additional benefits, such as:

✦ Decreased pain and stiffness.

✦ Stronger muscles and bones.

✦ Increased energy.

✦ Better quality of life.

✦ Weight control.

✦ Improved physical and mental health.

✦ Stress reduction.

Physical activity is safe and beneficial for most people. If you are not sure how much physical activity is safe for you, be sure to consult with a health-care professional. Remember to include the three main types of exercise outlined in Chapters 10, 11, and 12.

**A healthy diet and physical activity are
the keys to a healthy lifestyle.**

Start slowly and gradually increase your activity, remembering to practice the two-hour pain rule. Try to accumulate thirty minutes of activity on most days. You don't need to do all of the activity at one time. You can break up your exercise routine into ten-minute sessions, spread over the day. Increase your activity as your body grows accustomed to your new lifestyle. If you have an exercise program prescribed by a therapist, for a specific joint problem or muscle group, be sure to follow that program and include it in your routine.

You may want to make a weekly schedule that builds exercise into your day so that you can balance rest and activity. An example is provided in Table 16.3.

How Can I Develop an Exercise Habit?

Here are some suggestions to help you on the road to becoming more physically active:

✦ Build physical activity into your daily routine.

Table 16.3
Schedule for Physical Activity

Sunday	Stretching and range-of-motion exercises	Walk to church and back (ten minutes each way)		Strengthening exercises for arms
Monday	Do laundry	Aquafit class (forty minutes)		Walk around the block
Tuesday	Stretching and range-of-motion exercises	Clean the bathroom	Walk in the park (summer); mall walking group (winter)	Leg-strengthening exercises
Wednesday	Clean lower shelves in kitchen	Walk to the store and back (fifteen minutes each way)	Work in garden	Tai chi class (thirty minutes)
Thursday	Stretching and range-of-motion exercises	Aquafit class (forty minutes)		Do leg-strengthening exercises while watching TV
Friday	Grocery shopping	Walk around block (fifteen minutes total)	Vacuum living room	Do hand and arm exercises
Saturday	Mop kitchen floor	Leg-strengthening exercises	Ride bicycle to and from park (fifteen minutes each way)	Walk to friend's for dinner (ten minutes each way)

✦ Continue to do the activities you do now. Ask yourself: Can I do them more often?

✦ Start new activities slowly, and stretch frequently.

✦ Move around more often.

✦ Find a friend to encourage you.

✦ Find activities that you enjoy, such as nature walks, gardening, swimming, or dancing.

✦ Join a class in your community.

✦ Ask for suggestions from health-care professionals, community centers, and friends.

If you need more ideas about what activities you might enjoy, get more information from your health-care provider, the library, a community center, or your friends. Remember—the longer you sit, the harder it will be to get up and get going!

MANAGING STRESS AND KEEPING YOUR BALANCE

Stress arises from everyday life events such as interpersonal relationships, workplace pressures, and worries about things that may or may not happen. People with arthritis or related conditions such as fibromyalgia have the same life stresses as anyone else. In addition, they have the stress of managing pain, stiffness, and decreased energy. You may need to make changes in your lifestyle or give up activities that you really enjoy because of the effects of your arthritis. Life roles such as parenting, employment, and social activities may also change. All of this can be upsetting and stressful. Learning to recognize and deal with stress can make the changes easier to accept.

Understanding what stress is and how it affects the symptoms of arthritis can help you to decrease the negative effects that stress can have on your body. As you learn to recognize the signs and examine the things in your life that cause stress, you can take control and practice stress-management techniques. In this way, you can establish a more balanced approach to life and its challenges.

How Does Stress Affect My Body?

Your body reacts to stress by releasing chemicals into your blood that cause:

✦ An increase in your breathing rate.

✦ An increase in your blood pressure.

✦ A faster heartbeat.

✦ An increase in muscle tension.

If you are unable to deal with stress positively, tension builds up and can result in:

✦ Headache, neck, and back pain.

✦ Upset stomach.

✦ Disease flare-ups.

✦ Sleep problems.

✦ Change in appetite.

✦ A weakened immune system that can lead to other physical problems.

✦ Lack of sexual desire.

When you are stressed and your muscles become tense, increased pain and fatigue can limit your energy and your ability to carry out daily activities. You may become depressed. This is part of the cycle of pain described in Chapter 7. If you can understand and manage the stress, you can break the cycle. If you learn to manage the stress positively, the body can adjust and restore itself.

How Does Stress Affect My Emotions?

Stress can be described as a feeling that the outside world is impinging on you and creating the perception that you may not be able to cope. It can be thought of as an emergency signal that makes you "shift into a higher gear." A small amount of stress can be a good thing, because it helps you to do your best in situations like giving a speech, taking a test, or competing at a game. On the other hand, too much stress may result in a variety of emotional reactions, such as feelings of fear, anger, helplessness, or frustration.

Learn to recognize the signs of stress and the possible causes so that you can take steps to change things and take control. The following list contains suggestions for ways that you can limit stress in your life:

✦ Accept the fact that daily hassles and minor irritations are a part of everyday life.

✦ Realign your priorities. Ask yourself what is most important to you and what you can let go of, do differently, or delegate to someone else.

✦ Be kind to yourself. Take the time to relax. Practice deep breathing, learn relaxation techniques, or distract yourself by doing something that you enjoy

✦ Take time, each day, to "count your blessings." In this way, you can start to think more positively.

✦ Set goals; make a plan to reach them. Include recreational activities and time with friends in your daily plans. Review your goals regularly, and be flexible about the time you will need to accomplish them.

✦ Keep your sense of humor. If you are able to laugh at yourself, or at the situation, this is a great stress reliever.

✦ Spend your time doing the things in life that you value. Don't overcommit to unnecessary activities that stress you out. Learn to say no without feeling guilty.

Maintain a healthy balance in your life.

To strike a balance in your life, take a good look at your lifestyle, and think about the things that you find stressful and what it is that you can do to reduce or eliminate them. People vary in terms of their responses to different situations and what they perceive to be stressful. Some may like to keep busy and to be distracted by lots of activity. Others may wish to withdraw and be quiet and take things slowly. Recognizing which category you belong to will help you to manage stress. Changing your perception, or letting go of worries about what you can't change, can reshape your thinking and direct your energy toward positive action.

Having a Healthy Attitude

Some situations cannot be changed, and the only person whom you can change is yourself. Approach challenging situations and people with a positive attitude and you will be more successful than if you simply attempt to change things. If you can be flexible and keep an optimistic attitude, you can deal more easily with the difficulties. A negative attitude feeds on itself. If you persist in thinking, "This is only going to get worse," the situation generally does just that. Focusing on the positive (try saying to yourself, "Perhaps this is getting better") improves your ability to manage the stress.

Develop a healthy way of dealing with stressful situations. Put minor irritations like a late bus or a traffic jam in perspective. Ask yourself, "How important is this?" "Will I remember this in ten years; in five?" Looking objectively at the situation helps you to put it in perspective and manage it more effectively. Direct your attention to positive things you enjoy. Thinking about things that you enjoy and appreciate can help you to restore the balance.

One important way to cope with stress is to listen to your body's signals and learn to relax. Relaxation is more than just lying down and being quiet. There are a number of relaxation methods and processes that progressively calm your body and mind. Generally these methods take some practice, and not all relaxation methods work for everyone. You may need to try out different methods to find what is best for you. If you need help to learn how to relax, a mental-health professional such as a social worker or psychologist can help.

ADDRESSING SUBSTANCE-ABUSE ISSUES

How often do you hear people say that they are so stressed that they need a drink, a cigarette, or a pill to cope? These reactions are very common but are also very unhealthy. None of these substances will reduce stress; once their immediate effects wear off, the stress is still there, waiting for you. If you are a substance abuser or a smoker, analyze your use of these products, and be honest about whether you are using them to help yourself over rough spots. If you are, you need to make a plan to stop using these crutches.

Consuming alcohol moderately can help you to relax and enjoy social events, and drinking in moderation is not harmful to most people unless they have been advised by their doctor not to drink. There is even some evidence that alcohol can be beneficial to health when it is used wisely. However, if you use alcohol in order to cope with pain or to manage stress, this can be dangerous. You need to find healthier alternatives. It is important to discuss this with a health-care provider who can support you in your efforts to change dangerous habits.

If the effects of your arthritis and the stress in your life are overwhelming you, discuss this with your physician. If medications such as pain relievers, antidepressants, or tranquilizers are prescribed for you, be sure to follow the directions for dosage. Ask the doctor or pharmacist about their side effects and how long you should be on these medications. Exceeding the recommended dosage is dangerous and can lead to overdose. It is also dangerous to combine prescription medications with over-the-counter medications (e.g., taking a cold preparation such as a cough syrup, which may contain acetaminophen, along with a pain reliever such as Tylenol, which is acetaminophen). This is known as "layering" and can lead to overdosing. While medications can help with the effects of stress, relying on pharmaceuticals to solve your stress problems over the long run is not a prudent strategy.

Tobacco is highly addictive, and smoking is a habit that is extremely difficult to quit. Smoking moderately is not an option; quitting is the only healthy choice. People with rheumatoid arthritis who smoke tend to have more deformities and a positive "rheumatoid factor," which is an indicator of more severe disease. The benefits of quitting this habit are considerable and include improved heart and lung function, improved circulation, and better dental health. If you are a smoker, get all the help and support you need and quit smoking as soon as you can.

Be sure to seek out resources that can help you reach your targets. Reward yourself for even small successes. You are the manager of your arthritis, and you are in control of the choices you make. The web sites of both the Arthritis Foundation and The Arthritis Society have excellent information and pointers on adopting a healthy lifestyle. Accept the challenge to adopt a healthy lifestyle! Live well and enjoy your life more!

Looking Forward

This chapter has looked at the main lifestyle changes that you can make to effectively and positively deal with your arthritis and promote your own good health. Focusing on key lifestyle issues will help you maintain your health and wellness through the ups and downs of arthritis. Being well puts you in a better position to respond positively to medical interventions like new medications or potential surgical options. The following chapter addresses the important topic of surgery.

Chapter 17

Exploring Options for Joint Surgery

For the majority of individuals who suffer from arthritis, pain and inflammation can be treated effectively with medications. Equally important in arthritis management are exercise, joint protection, and energy conservation, as well as access to emotional and social support. However, for individuals who have severe, long-term arthritis, and whose joints and related structures are destroyed due to joint inflammation or degeneration, surgery may be the most viable option for relief. Individuals with osteoarthritis may need surgery for one or two joints; those with inflammatory arthritis may require surgery for several joints. This chapter discusses the different issues you should be aware of if you are considering joint surgery, as well as steps you can take to ensure the best possible results for any surgical treatment you may undergo.

The decision to pursue surgical options requires a team approach. The decision typically involves a primary-care physician, a rheumatologist or internist, the orthopedic surgeon who will perform the surgery, the physical or occupational therapists who will help with rehabilitation, and the most important team member—you, the patient. If possible, consult an orthopedic surgeon before damage and deformity have been established in the earlier stages of arthritis. This allows the surgeon to monitor changes and determine the most appropriate time for surgery, helping to ensure the best outcome. This chapter will provide you with the information you need to lead your health-care management team as you explore your surgical options.

**The decision to have surgery should involve
key members of the health-care team.**

NOW MORE THAN EVER

Over the past thirty years, great strides have been made in joint surgery and surgery on related structures. New and improved techniques have been developed, especially in the area of artificial replacement of joints, or arthroplasty. Now, a variety of metal alloys, high-density polymers, and ceramic materials are utilized to replace and resurface joints. It is currently possible for an artificial joint to last twelve or more years before requiring a revision (a procedure to replace a component of the artificial joint or to remove excess bone or scar tissue) or a complete replacement. In older patients, a new artificial joint may suffice for a lifetime.

**Great strides have been made in replacement
surgery for hip and knee joints.**

SHOULD I CONSIDER SURGERY?

Consider surgery if you experience one or more of the following problems:

✦ Pain associated with movement, weight-bearing, or resting that can be relieved only by narcotic drugs.

✦ Inability to perform normal activities of daily living, such as walking without aids, ascending or descending stairs, getting in and out of a car, manipulating common objects, dressing and undressing, and attending to personal hygiene.

✦ Difficulties at work that require reduced hours or that result in your inability to work altogether.

✦ Damage to a joint or its associated structures that results in severe loss of movement, joint instability, and gross joint misalignment.

Not everyone responds equally well to surgery. Some people are considered to be better candidates with a higher chance for a better outcome. Issues that will affect how likely a candidate you are for surgery include:

✦ General joint health; neighboring joints, or joints in the opposite limbs, must be in good condition to provide support in the early stages of surgical recovery.

✦ Body weight; excessive obesity is a contraindication for knee or hip joint replacement.

✦ Willingness to adhere to advice and recommendations of the treatment team.

✦ Ability to survive the surgery; patients in extremely poor health are at an especially high risk.

When Is Surgery Not Recommended?

The success of a surgical intervention will be compromised if any of the following conditions exist:

✦ Poor health. Poor health is often a factor for patients who have heart disease and may be at risk of developing life-threatening blood clots following surgery. Also at risk are: patients with severe respiratory problems that can limit the choice of anesthetics used; patients who have severe arthritis of the neck who are unable to move the head and neck freely; and patients who may require the use of special tubes to administer the anesthetic.

✦ Active infection of joints or neighboring structures.

✦ Inadequate bone structure.

✦ Inability to move the limbs due to paralysis.

✦ Obesity due to underlying disease, such as diabetes.

✦ Emotional instability.

People who are not overweight and have established good wellness habits are usually very good candidates for joint surgery.

WHAT TYPES OF SURGERIES ARE COMMON FOR ARTHRITIS PATIENTS?

Surgery is used to achieve two main objectives: relief of pain and improvement or restoration of joint function. Although arthroplasty, also known as joint replacement, is the most common type of surgery for arthritis patients, surgery for arthritis is not confined to the joints or the use of artificial joints. Surgery may also be indicated to correct the alignment of tendons, relieve pressure on nerves (as in carpal tunnel syndrome), and remove bursae and nodules. The most common procedures are arthroplasty, debridement, arthrodesis, synovectomy, osteotomy, tendon transfer or repair, nerve decompression, bursectomy, and nodule resection.

✦ **Arthroplasty** is the replacement of a damaged joint with an artificial joint. Arthroplasties can be performed on most joints; however, they mainly are performed on hip, knee, or shoulder joints. Arthroplasties are needed when a joint is completely damaged and extremely painful during rest and activity. The bone structure above and below the joint must be sound to permit good adhesion of the artificial parts, and the patient should have good control over joint movement. In some cases in which the damage is confined to only one of the joint surfaces, a partial arthroplasty may be performed. Figure 17.1 illustrates a total knee replacement or arthroplasty.

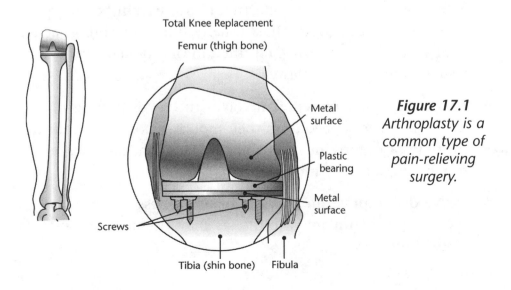

Total Knee Replacement

Femur (thigh bone)

Metal surface

Plastic bearing

Metal surface

Screws

Tibia (shin bone)   Fibula

Figure 17.1 Arthroplasty is a common type of pain-relieving surgery.

✦ **Debridement** involves cleaning up a joint by removing cartilage fragments or debris, loose bone, or thickened and inflamed synovial membranes.

✦ **Arthrodesis** is the fusion of two or more joints to permanently restrict joint movement. It is commonly performed on the spinal column in the presence of spinal instability or intractable pain, or when pressure on nerves issuing from the spinal column is in the process of leading to paralysis. Arthrodesis is sometimes performed as an alternative to arthroplasty on limb joints, or when arthroplasty has failed. Joints in close proximity to the arthrodesis should have a reasonable amount of movement in order to compensate for the loss of movement in the arthrodesed joint.

✦ **Synovectomy** is the removal of synovial membrane to protect articular cartilage or tendons from substances in the degraded synovium that can cause damaging biochemical reactions.

✦ **Osteotomy** is the practice of cutting the bone immediately above or below a joint, then allowing it to heal in a more favorable position in order to redistribute the weight-bearing pressure on damaged joints. It is usually done on young, active adults who have extensive destruction of articular cartilage, as a substitute for arthroplasty.

✦ **Tendon transfer or repair** involves the repositioning of tendons that have slipped from their moorings, or are frayed, and in some cases torn, due to damaging biochemical reactions or roughening of bony tunnels.

✦ **Nerve decompression** provides relief of pressure on nerves in the vicinity of inflamed joints, as may occur in the case of carpal tunnel syndrome.

✦ **Bursectomy** is the removal of inflamed bursa. Recall that a bursa is a fluid-filled sac lodged between two moving surfaces that is designed to remove friction.

✦ **Nodule resection** is the removal of arthritic nodules that are painful and unsightly.

WHICH JOINTS RECEIVE PRIORITY FOR SURGERY?

Patients with inflammatory arthritis may require surgery for several joints. Some joints are operated on before others in order to achieve the best results. The order of priorities, starting with the most important, are listed below.

✦ The joints of the neck (cervical spine) take priority if they are unstable and likely to damage the spinal cord.

✦ The large joints of the lower limb—hips, knees, or ankles—are also high on the list.

✦ If the joints of the upper limb—shoulders, elbows, wrists, or fingers—are severely damaged, and the damage would make the use of walking aids following lower-limb surgery difficult, then these upper-body limbs will be a higher priority than the lower-limb joints.

✦ The dominant arm or leg is given priority over the non-dominant arm or leg. The dominant arm, used frequently for fine or gross movements, will most likely receive an arthroplasty, while the non-dominant arm or leg, used for holding or stabilizing activities, is more likely to receive an arthrodesis.

HOW SHOULD I PREPARE FOR SURGERY?

In general, physically fit people recover more quickly after surgery than those who are unfit. This is especially true in people who undergo surgery to their large joints, such as the hips or knees. Because most patients with arthritis are often unfit—due to the disease and its effects on physical function—a pre-operative fitness program is important. Arthritis affecting the upper joints in the neck can be life-threatening or could lead to paralysis and therefore may require urgent surgery. Surgery to other damaged joints or structures, however, is usually elective, allowing patients and the surgical team ample time to prepare for the surgery.

**Fit people recover more quickly after surgery
than those who are unfit.**

A pre-operative group program is usually offered that typically addresses many of the following concerns:

✦ **Education.** An orthopedic surgeon and/or a physical therapist usually provide patient education. They explain the need for surgery, the importance of preparing for surgery, what to expect immediately following surgery, and what to expect in the long term.

✦ **Pain Control.** Instructions are offered regarding pain management following surgery.

✦ **General Fitness.** An exercise fitness program is essential before surgery, as the pain and disability resulting from arthritis can be very debilitating. Patients who are fit before their surgery recover faster after their surgery. Typical pre-operative exercise programs focus on endurance exercise, such as walking, cycling, low-impact aerobics, or water aerobics.

+ **Mobility Exercises.** Joint stiffness is often the bane of people with arthritis. The range of movement in the joints close to the site of surgery must be maintained or increased by means of mobilizing exercises. The strength and mobility of the joints of the opposite limb and those of nearby limbs must also be maintained to help with ambulation and the activities of daily living during recovery.

+ **Strengthening Exercises.** The muscles moving an arthritic joint become weak due to pain and disuse. Pre-operative strengthening exercises involving these muscles will speed their recovery following surgery. For lower-limb surgery, the muscles of the opposite limb and the muscles of the upper limbs must be strengthened to prepare the patient for walking with crutches or canes following surgery.

+ **Circulatory Exercises.** Patients who may be confined to bed following surgery must be made aware before surgery of the need to maintain the flow of blood in the lower limbs. This prevents the potential for life-threatening, deep-vein thrombosis (DVT). Deep-vein thrombosis occurs when a blood clot develops in the large veins of the lower body and can be avoided with hourly foot, ankle, and knee exercises to keep the blood in the deep veins flowing.

+ **Breathing Exercises.** The general anesthetic given during surgery tends to reduce the movement of cilia (little hairs) in the air passages of the respiratory system. When cilia move less, mucus can accumulate and plug air passages. Patients should be taught deep-breathing exercises and productive coughing techniques so air continues to flow in and out of the lungs and the air passages are kept clear of mucus. If the air passages are plugged with mucus, part of the lung or the whole lung may collapse.

✦ **Assistive Devices.** Depending on the type of surgery performed, patients must be shown how to use a number of assistive devices to help with their post-surgical rehabilitation. They also may need to learn new methods of going about their daily activities post-surgery. Instruction may be needed in how to use walking aids, such as a walker or crutches; how to sit and rise from a raised toilet seat; how to enter and exit a shower or bathtub; how to put on and take off splints that support the site of the operation; how to use various assistive devices to dress and undress; and how to eat or drink using specially designed cups, forks, knives, and spoons.

Circulatory and breathing exercises are important following surgery to prevent life-threatening complications.

LIFE AFTER SURGERY

The two main objectives of arthritis surgery are the relief of pain and improvement of function. Ironically, even surgery that is undergone to ultimately reduce pain can be a major source of pain in the early stages of recovery.

For patients who have a joint replaced, pain and discomfort can be heightened further, because physical exercise to restore joint mobility and muscle strength must begin a day or two after surgery. Aggressive pain management before exercise using narcotic agents is crucial at this stage. Pain that is not managed well and completely at this early stage can persist and become increasingly difficult to treat.

After surgery, patients will likely stay in the hospital a few days and receive physical therapy while they recover. Immediately following surgery, a patient will be started on a routine of foot and ankle exercises to maintain blood flow and prevent life-threatening blood clots. Deep-breathing exercises and coughing are also crtical at this stage. These exercises will maintain lung expansion and help clear air passages that can become plugged with mucus.

A general exercise program for the non-operated limbs also must be initiated to keep patients fit for walking and normal activities. This fitness regime usually consists of frequent isometric presses in bed. Patients will be shown methods to safely sit up in bed and slowly transfer body weight from lying to sitting, from sitting to standing, and from standing to walking.

One or two days following surgery, the physical therapist will begin specific exercises on the operated limb or joint that are designed to strengthen muscles and mobilize joints that are swollen and painful to move. Pain-relieving drugs may be given before each exercise session in the early days. When the surgical wound has healed more, vigorous exercises are begun, and the patient is taught how to slowly resume activities of daily living. If possible, exercise in a therapeutic pool can be very helpful, as the buoyancy of the water allows movement without the stressing effect of gravity.

If the operated site is immobilized to permit healing, pain management using ice packs, in addition to narcotics, is equally important following immobilization. Like painkillers, ice packs are key to ensuring that exercise, which is crucial at this stage, is better tolerated. In these cases, exercises should be started immediately after the restraint has been removed.

Upon discharge, patients will require physical therapy at home or in an outpatient facility to continue the process of rehabilitation and recovery.

After-Care of Arthroplasties

Arthroplasties (artificial joint replacements) are the most common form of arthritis surgery and the most difficult to perform. Of these, hip and knee arthroplasties are performed the most frequently and deserve special attention here. To avoid serious complications from hip or knee arthroplasty and to hasten recovery, pay special attention to the following :

✦ **The Wound.** Immediately after surgery, the wound will be monitored by the attending physician and hospital staff. Watch for warning signs of infection, including abnormal redness, increasing warmth, swelling, or unusual pain. Report any injury to the joint immediately.

✦ **Walking.** A walker is easier and safer to use than a cane during the first few weeks. Younger patients can manage well on crutches. The use of a walker or crutches reduces the chance of soft tissues separating. After six weeks, a cane may be used.

✦ **Sleeping.** To avoid dislocating your hip after a hip replacement keep your legs apart when you are lying on your back, and place a pillow between your knees when you are lying on your side. With a new knee, you may sleep in any position.

✦ **Seating.** Avoid soft, low chairs or sofas; choose firm, higher chairs with stable arms that allow you to ease into sitting and standing positions. Avoid crossing your legs or rotating your hips when you are sitting or lying down. Standard-height toilet seats tend to compress joints in extreme positions. Use a raised toilet seat—two to four inches higher than the standard height—or use a toilet-seat extender.

✦ **Driving.** Driving a car with an automatic shift is generally permissible after the first six weeks. Adjust the seat as far back as possible to prevent compression of your hips. Drive carefully, as your reaction time will be slower. Avoid extreme positions when you get in and out of a car. Avoid cars with very low seats.

◆ **Work.** If you have a strenuous job that requires a lot of walking and heavy lifting, you will need three to six months before you return to work. Avoid lifting loads heavier than twenty-five pounds. With a desk job, you may be able to return to work after four weeks.

◆ **At Home.** Arrange the furniture to provide ample room to navigate with a walker or crutches. Remove small, slippery floor rugs, as they can increase your risk of falling.

◆ **Activities.** Future activities are generally limited to those that do not put you at risk of injuring the replaced joints. Avoid sports that involve running or contact in favor of less dangerous sports such as golf, bowling, and swimming. Swimming is the ideal form of exercise, because it improves muscle strength and endurance without exerting any pressure or stress on replaced joints.

◆ **Risk of Infection.** Alert your doctor or dentist that you have an artificial joint. These joints are at risk of infection by the bacteria introduced via invasive procedures such as surgery, dental or gum work, and urologic or endoscoping procedures, as well as from infections elsewhere in the body. Take a high dose of antibiotics before, during, and after such procedures in order to prevent infection of the replaced joint.

◆ **Re-operation.** Infrequently, patients with joint replacements may require a second operation years later. The second operation may be necessary because of loosening, fracture, or other complications. Re-operations are generally not as successful as the original operation and carry a higher risk of complications.

Looking Forward

In the past three decades, advances in arthritis surgery has brought relief to millions of sufferers. While the short-term risks of surgery are often high, the long-term benefits typically far outweigh these initial costs. Hopefully, the content in this chapter has provided you with the information you need to make important decisions about the surgical options that many arthritis patients face. Earlier chapters in the book armed you with information about additionally proven treatment regimes, such as new medications, therapy options, and exercise programs. The last chapter of the book describes some common *unproven* therapies in an effort to help you distinguish which alternative remedies may be harmful or ineffective, and which are worth exploring further.

Chapter 18

Exercising Caution About Cures and Testimonials

Patients with chronic diseases such as arthritis are bombarded by claims about cures, old and new. These cures and claims promising to miraculously restore good health and enjoyment of life are found everywhere in newspapers, on radio and television, and more recently on the Internet. But media outlets and the Internet are often not the sole source of the onslaught; you may also hear about wonder cures from well-intentioned friends, co-workers, and relatives.

In the early part of the twentieth century, medical science was not well versed in the various forms of arthritis. Arthritis was considered an unavoidable consequence of aging and therefore beyond the influence of the average physician or the reach of medical investigations. A better awareness of arthritis in all of its various forms came about during the Second World War, when many young army recruits were rejected on the basis of back pain that was subsequently recognized to be ankylosing spondylitis. Since that time, many different forms of arthritis have been identified—forms that affect males and females of all ages, including children. This discovery has led to thousands of scientific studies seeking a treatment gold standard for each of the different diagnostic categories. Today, health scientists and health-care workers can recommend a myriad of forms of treatment, including pharmaceuticals, surgery, and physical rehabilitation. And thanks to the efforts of research scientists, the efficacy of these established treatments is backed up by hard scientific evidence.

In this chapter, we will explore the way in which researchers discover and test treatments for arthritis. After we have established what makes a treatment legitimate in the eyes of the mainstream medical community, we will look into the claims of so-called "alternative" treatment plans and practitioners. By doing so, we hope to provide you with some basic guidelines to apply as you attempt to make personal choices in the face of the glut of information and testimonials.

HOW DO HEALTH SCIENTISTS KNOW THAT A NEW TREATMENT WILL WORK?

The search for new treatments is labor-intensive. Scientists search for years to find a pharmaceutical agent, a specific treatment, or a surgical procedure that may have treatment potential. They first experiment on cells and tissues in their laboratories, then they experiment on animals, and finally they test treatments on humans. Even after all of the preliminary research in labs and on animal subjects, it may take an additional five years or more of intensive work with human subjects to prove a treatment's benefits. The process is summarized in Figure 18.1.

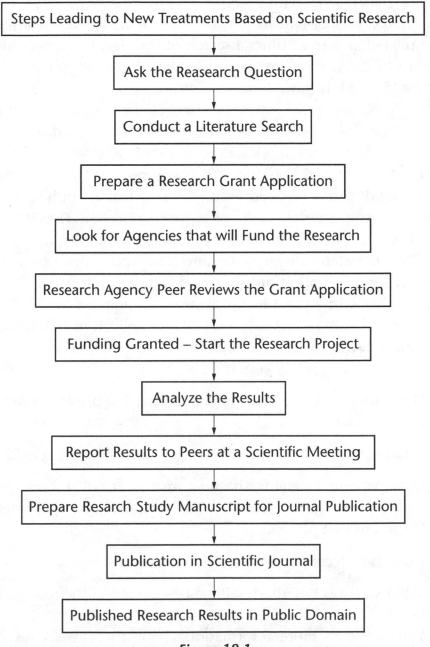

Figure 18.1
*Numerous steps are taken by scientists to determine
the efficacy of arthritis treatments.*

The search starts with a simple research question; for example, *Does aerobic exercise improve physical function in rheumatoid arthritis?* The next step is to conduct a search in the health-sciences litera- ture to find out what has been written on the subject. If others have addressed the question in a satisfactory manner, then the sci- entists typically move on to another research topic. Sometimes, even when the question may have been well answered by others, it is useful to try and duplicate the methods of previous studies to find out if new studies produce the same results. Through repeat- ed testing of the same hypothesis, different teams can help to val- idate or invalidate the results of previous research. The literature search alone may take three to six months to complete.

The next steps are to determine a protocol, describe it in a research grant application, and find a research-funding agency that might be interested in the answer to the question. To secure funding, scientists are asked to create an application that includes key information about their proposed research protocol. They must inform the agency about:

✦ How subjects are selected and how many subjects are needed for the study.

✦ What treatment and treatment safeguards will be offered.

✦ How patients receiving the new treatment will be compared with another group receiving no treatment or an alternative treatment or a placebo.

✦ How the effects of the treatments will be assessed.

✦ What statistical methods will be used to assess the results.

You can read more information about the various research processes in Chapter 5. The funding agency sends the protocol out for peer review to determine the merits of the proposed research. If a researcher succeeds in the competition for limited funds he or she is "off to the races." This protocol preparation stage and funding may take more than a year to complete.

**It takes time to determine the effectiveness
of any new arthritis treatment.**

Next, the lead scientist will gather a research team and conduct the study. It is important that the team do so without any deviations from the agreed-upon study protocol. It is also important that the team members document all of their activities so that the research results can be duplicated and verified. The patient safeguards built into the study protocol will help protect participants against any ill effects of the experiment. This process may take two to three years to complete.

Once the study is complete, the researcher will want to analyze and assess the results and then report them—whether the results are positive, negative, or show no change—first to his or her peers at a scientific meeting, where researchers are certain to receive a critical review and feedback. Then a study manuscript is written and submitted to a scientific journal. The journal editors will send the article to other scientists, who are experts in the topic of the research, for peer review and comments. Once the study is accepted for publication, it is in the public domain, which means that it is accessible to anyone who chooses to read it. This process may take a year or more, depending on the timing of the scientific meeting and the queue of articles in the appropriate journal.

If the study concludes that the new treatment is better than an old treatment or better than no treatment or the placebo, *and* that it can be provided at a reasonable cost, then the new treatment is deemed successful. If the benefits are the same as an old treatment, but the costs are higher, then the old treatment remains the treatment of choice. If test subjects who received the new treatment fare no better than those who received no treatment or the placebo, then the new treatment has failed.

**Careful research is the best guarantee
that treatments are safe and effective.**

Hundreds of thousands of health scientists worldwide are trying to answer different questions using the process just described. This kind of research is labor-intensive and comes at a high cost, but it is the best guarantee that the treatment you are being offered is effective and safe. The process is not foolproof, but it has the potential to benefit patients in the majority of cases. *Evidence-based practice*—health-care practice in which treatment choices are based on scientific evidence—has become the norm among legitimate health-care professionals. To prevent fraud, the standards for treatment methods have been tightened, and large groups of scientists are collecting and evaluating scientific articles on specific treatments in order to firmly establish treatment standards that best benefit patients.

COMPLEMENTARY AND ALTERNATIVE HEALTH CARE (CAHC)

Complementary and alternative health care (CAHC) is a term used to refer to a group of diverse medical and health-care systems, practices, and products that are not presently considered to be part of conventional health care. Conventional health care for arthritis is evidence-based practice that is conducted by holders of doctors of medicine or osteopathy degrees, and by licensed applied-health professionals, such as nurses, physical therapists, occupational therapists, and dietitians. Some practitioners of conventional health care are also practitioners of CAHC.

Many CAHC therapies for arthritis are heavily advertised and make attractive claims. Often these claims are based on personal experiences or testimonials. Remember that a personal anecdote is not the same as research; it is important to find out whether any high-quality scientific research has been done on a CAHC therapy before you decide to try it. None of the CAHC therapies discussed in this book have been proven to be of benefit for arthritis using the rigorous process described in the previous section of this chapter. Efforts are being made to subject CAHC therapies to the same standards of scientific research used in conventional health care, but these efforts are currently weak and, on the whole, ineffective.

Why Do Some People With Arthritis Turn to CAHC Therapies?

There are many reasons why some people with arthritis resort to CAHC therapies, including the following:

✦ Conventional treatment is not working as well as hoped.

✦ People want greater relief of symptoms and disability.

✦ There are problems with side effects of prescribed conventional drugs and treatments.

✦ People resolve to take any measures available to reduce some of the pain, discomfort, and stress that come from living with a chronic illness.

✦ There is a belief that CAHC therapies are safer and more "natural."

✦ There is pressure from the widespread advertising and exaggerated claims of many CAHC products.

**People may turn to CAHC therapies when they
are frustrated by other treatment options.**

Issues to Keep in Mind When Considering CAHC Therapies

If you have arthritis and are thinking of using a CAHC therapy, the following are some important points to keep in mind:

✦ To get effective treatment, it is crucial that a well-trained health practitioner who has a conventional health education and experience with arthritis patients provide a diagnosis for you.

✦ Proven conventional treatment for arthritis should not be replaced with a CAHC treatment that is unproven.

✦ Tell all conventional health-care providers about any and all supplements, drugs (prescription, over-the-counter, or "alternative"), or other therapies that you are using or considering. Prescribed drugs may need to be adjusted if you are also using CAHC therapies. Medications and supplements can interact with drugs (even if they are non-prescription "alternative" or "natural" substances). This interaction can affect how your body responds both to your normal medication and to the new CAHC treatment.

✦ Governments do not regulate supplements in the same way they do conventional medications, and there is very little oversight on labeling in the supplements industry. The ingredients list that you see on the label of a supplement may not reflect what is actually in the bottle. Some herbal supplements have been found to be contaminated with heavy metals or prescription drugs, and some have been found to have much more or much less of certain ingredients than their labels report.

✦ The claims for many CAHC therapies can be exaggerated and deceptively attractive, ranging from enhanced well-being to miraculous cures for chronic conditions.

✦ Women who are pregnant or nursing, or people who are thinking of using CAHC to treat a child, should use extra caution and be sure to consult their health-care provider.

Government agencies do not regulate most "natural" remedies and supplements like they do conventional health-care treatments.

WHAT ABOUT HERBAL REMEDIES?

It is easy to forget that the modern pharmaceutical industry has its roots in the ancient art of botanizing. Botanizing is the label that early apothecaries gave to the activity of collecting plants that have useful medical properties. Even the first synthetic blockbuster drugs—Bayer aspirin, digoxin, and heroin—were simply minor modifications of molecules extracted from the willow bark, foxglove plants, and poppyseed pods, respectively.

People in much of the world still rely on herbs for medicines. Used correctly, herbs can be helpful. The problem that we encounter with herbal medicines is limited research about what truly works, and what does not. There are also issues regarding quality control for these products that are not the result of scientific research or standard production methods. For example, different producers of herbal medicines often recommend different dosages of the same product, and they report different claims for the herb's beneficial effects for a host of chronic and sometimes incurable diseases.

Despite the fact that herbals are widely used, there is little high-quality scientific evidence available to determine if and how patients can safely use these products. Recognizing this need, The National Center for Complementary and Alternative Medicine—a branch of the National Institutes of Health—was established in 1998 in the United States to fund and promote scientific studies of the effectiveness of herbal medicines and other alternative hands-on treatments, or treatment devices. While the quality of this research has improved over time, many research studies do not thoroughly describe the herbal medicine being studied. This is significant, because herbal medicines are natural products, and the active ingredient can vary in potency due to many factors, including how and where the product was grown, how it was manufactured, the purity and strength of the ingredients, and the product's shelf life. There are also no standards of manufacture, and the same herbals may vary in strength and purity among competing manufacturers.

Individuals who are desperate to find a cure, or who believe only in "natural" remedies, are easy targets for peddlers of unproven herbal products. Promoters of herbal medicines and other CAHC therapies for the treatment of arthritis play to a captive audience. Patients who are ill-informed about scientific evidence, or those who are obsessed with natural remedies, are easy targets for promoters of herbal medicines.

Herbals are widely used, particularly by women sixty-five years of age and older. Information from one survey in the United States shows that more than 25 percent of older women take some form of herbal or other "natural" products. Frequently used products are glucosamine for arthritis, garlic for elevated cholesterol, and ginkgo biloba for memory enhancement. Perhaps the main reason why herbal medicines are so popular is the misconception that, because they are "natural," they are entirely safe.

Tell your health-care provider about any "natural" supplements you may be taking.

Even patients who are under a conventional physician's care and receiving scientifically proven treatments often indulge in unproven treatments for "extra insurance." This is risky, because quite often a medically prescribed drug can interact with an herbal supplement if taken at the same time, with serious consequences. For example, ginkgo biloba may interact with warfarin (coumadin), a frequently prescribed blood thinner, putting the patient at increased risk of bleeding. St. John's wort, taken in combination with some forms of prescribed antidepressants, may make patients confused and agitated. And echinacea, an herb that is supposed to stimulate the immune system, should not be used by people who have rheumatoid arthritis or lupus with a compromised immune system. Much more research is required to better understand these possible interactions.

It is important to talk to your physician before you start taking an herbal medicine. Survey data show that more than 50 percent of people who take an herbal medicine do not alert their physician. This may be because patients feel uncomfortable talking about CAHC therapies with their physician. As part of a medication review, physicians and pharmacists now are beginning to routinely ask patients about their use of herbal or other natural products. It is important for patients to bring all of their medications to their physician, including natural-health products and over-the-counter medications, whether taken by mouth, in the form of a suppository, or applied to the skin.

In summary, not much good research is available regarding the effectiveness and safety of herbal medicines that people commonly try for arthritis. In the United States, the U.S. Food and Drug Administration regulates these supplements and herbals as "food products" rather than as drugs, in spite of the fact that these supplements used for medicinal purposes can have effects and side effects as powerful as those of prescribed drugs. For this reason, use supplements and herbs only under the supervision of your physician or pharmacist. The following review of herbal therapies has been excerpted from a review conducted by the National Center for Complimentary and Alternative Medicine (NCCAM) in the United States. The publication is not copyrighted and is in the public domain. You can find out more about the NCCAM and its findings at http://nccam.nih.gov/.

Safety Information About Selected Herbal Supplements

It is important to be as informed as possible about the safety of any supplement you are considering. For many herbs, untested or anecdotal information is available from a long history of botanical use outside conventional medicine. Recently, some promising evidence-based studies are being conducted in the United States and Canada on herbals and supplements. The objective of these more rigorous, regulated investigations is to find out more about herbal composition, safety, function, and the specific conditions that the herbs may affect. The following describes some of the features of common herbs and supplements that have traditonally been used to treat arthritis.

✦ **Thunder God Vine (TGV).** TGV is a perennial vine native to China. Preparations made from the skinned root of TGV have been used in traditional Chinese medicine to treat inflammatory and autoimmune diseases. Preliminary studies in the United States using TGV on twenty-one rheumatoid arthritis patients have shown improvement in symptoms and physical functioning. However, the sample of patients was very small. Longer and larger studies are needed to confirm these findings. The leaves, the flowers, the main stem, and the skin covering the root of TGV are poisonous and could be fatal. There are no consistent, high-quality preparations of TGV in the United States and Canada and preparations made in China are probably not safe or effective. Long-term use in women can cause osteoporosis (thinning of bones); other side effects may include stomach upset, diarrhea, skin rash, hair loss, and changes in menstruation.

Herbals can be very powerful—just because a substance comes from a plant does not necessarily mean that it is gentle.

✦ **Gamma-linolenic acid (GLA).** GLA is a fatty acid found in the oils of some plant seeds, including evening primrose, borage, and black current. GLA can be used by the body to make substances that reduce inflammation. Several studies of GLA have been conducted, but inadequate research design makes it difficult to draw conclusions from the research. Some studies indicate that GLA provides some relief of pain, morning stiffness, and joint tenderness. Side effects of these oils can include nausea, diarrhea, soft stool, intestinal gas, and stomach bloating. GLA can also interact with prescription medication and affect certain conditions. It may increase the risk of bruising and bleeding in people taking blood-thinning drugs, such as aspirin, coumadin, clopidogrel, and NSAIDs. It can also interact with the psychiatric drugs phenothiazine, chlorpromazine, and prochlorperazine.

✦ **Fish oil.** Fish oil contains high amounts of fatty acids. The human body can use fish oil (like GLA) to make substances that can reduce inflammation. Several studies have shown that it can reduce the number of tender joints, morning stiffness, and the need for NSAIDs. Further studies are needed to determine the effective dosage and the length of treatment that benefit patients the most, and whether a placebo effect is at work. High doses of fish oil can increase the risk of bleeding or affect the time it takes for the blood to clot in some individuals. If you are taking drugs that affect bleeding, or you are going to have surgery, this is of special concern. Fish-oil supplements can interact with medications for high blood pressure; when taken in conjunction with high-blood-pressure medications, they can lower the blood pressure too much. People who decide to use fish oil should look for products made from fish with lower levels of mercury. Fish oil from sharks, swordfish, and mackerel is known to have high levels of mercury. Check with the manufacturers to find out from what type of fish the oil has been derived. Fish-liver oil, a related by product, contains vitamin A in higher amounts than the recommended daily dose. The side effects of ingesting fish oil include a fishy aftertaste, belching, stomach distress, and nausea.

+ **Glucosamine and chondroitin**. These are popular dietary supplements for treating arthritis. They are sold separately, in combination with each other, or in combination with other drugs. Glucosamine is a substance found in the fluid around the joints. It can also be obtained from the shells of shrimp, crab, and lobsters, or it can be manufactured in the laboratory. The body uses glucosamine to repair joint cartilage lining the bone ends. Chondroitin is a substance found in the cartilage around joints. It is obtained from sharks and cattle. Animal studies show that these two substances produce anti-inflammatory effects. In humans, glucosamine and chondroitin have been studied only in osteoarthritis and were shown to provide only modest benefit.

Glucosamine appears to be safe for most people. However, it can exacerbate the symptoms of asthma through an allergic reaction. It can also cause higher blood sugar and insulin levels in people with diabetes; those who decide to use it need to carefully monitor their blood sugar. Glucosamine can also possibly decrease the effectiveness of certain medications, such as acetaminophen, some anti-cancer drugs, and some anti-diabetes drugs. Side effects include mild stomach upset, nausea, sleepiness, a skin reaction, or headache.

Chondroitin appears to be safe for most people. However, it may possibly worsen asthma, blood-clotting disorders, and prostate cancer. Side effects of chondroitin include stomach pain and nausea; less commonly, you may experience diarrhea, constipation, and problems with your heart.

+ **Valerian.** Valerian is an herb used for sleep problems and anxiety disorders. Because sleep problems are common among patients with arthritis, many look to CAHC remedies for sleep assistance. Valerian has also been recommended to treat muscle and joint pain. Evidence suggests that it helps people with insomnia, but no studies have been done on arthritis patients to suggest that valerian helps with muscle and joint pain. There is no evidence on how long it is safe to take valerian and which dose to use. Valerian should not be taken with sedative drugs or herbs, as it may increase the sedative effect. Use caution when driving or operating heavy machinery when you are taking valerian. People taking antifungal drugs, statins, or certain anti-arrhythmia drugs should not take valerian. It is also not safe for patients with liver disorders.

✦ **Ginger, curcumin, boswellia, feverfew.** These four botanicals are commonly marketed with claims to benefit arthritis pain. They have been used historically to treat inflammatory conditions and are currently undergoing scientific trials. Ginger can cause stomach upset, diarrhea, and mouth and throat irritation. It is not recommended for people who have bleeding disorders, heart conditions, or diabetes. Curcumin can cause stomach problems, nausea, and diarrhea. It could compound the effects of other drugs or herbs that slow blood clotting. It can cause gallbladder contractions and should not be used by people with gallbladder disease or stones. Boswellia can cause stomach upset and pain, nausea, and diarrhea. It is not known whether boswellia interacts with any drugs, supplements, or diseases and conditions. Feverfew appears to be safe for short-term use, but the safety of long-term use is unknown; it can cause allergic reactions in people who are allergic to the daisy family. Side effects may include diarrhea and other stomach problems. Chewing fresh leaves of feverfew may cause mouth irritation and sores. Feverfew might interact with medications broken down by the liver and increase the action of drugs that slow blood clotting. Pregnant women should not take feverfew.

SPECIAL DIETS

Many people with arthritis are interested in how foods may affect their symptoms. Examples of foods that are believed to possibly worsen the symptoms of arthritis are the nightshade family of plants (white potatoes, tomatoes, eggplant, and pepper), dairy products, citrus fruits, acidic foods, sweets, coffee, and animal protein. There is no strong, reproducible evidence that any foods or diets have a specific role in causing or curing arthritis. It is important for people with arthritis to eat a healthy, balanced diet. If one or more foods are eliminated from the diet, it is possible to miss key nutrients and not get enough calories. It is important to discuss any major dietary changes with your health-care provider or a registered dietitian.

In the past, fasting regimes were tried by patients with rheumatoid arthritis and were found effective in reducing the symptoms of inflammation and pain. This effect occurs because fasting suppresses the immune system. However, continuous fasting is detrimental to life, and its practice cannot be justified.

**People with arthritis should eat
a healthy, balanced diet.**

A true food allergy may exist in a small percentage of patients. Many people think that they have food allergies when they do not have them or when they suffer from food intolerances. If you believe that you have a serious food allergy, discuss your concerns with your physician. He or she can test you and, if you are allergic, work with you to develop a diet that allows you to avoid allergens and still meet all of your nutritional requirements.

Various theories abound about how foods may relate to arthritis. Some proposed links include the following:

✦ The food you eat, and how the digestive system handles those foods, is known to affect the immune system. Because certain forms of arthritis, such as rheumatoid arthritis, are diseases of the immune system, a connection between diet and the immune system has been proposed.

✦ Certain fats (mostly from animal sources, but also from corn and sunflower oils) are known to break down into substances that can cause inflammation in the body.

✦ The medications used to treat inflammatory arthritis may affect the way a person's digestive system handles foods.

✦ Arthritis can affect a person's ability to prepare and eat food, leading to nutritional problems that can accentuate health problems.

Food is the fuel that your body needs to keep you as healthy as you can be. The better the fuel you use, the better you will feel. It is important for everyone to eat a healthy, balanced diet, and this is especially true for arthritis patients. Making sure that you eat a varied diet and get the right amount of calories should be a top priority for you every day. Please see Chapter 16 for more information on how to choose healthy foods in the right amounts for yourself. And just as you should ask your physician about any "natural" supplements you may want to take, you should consult with health-care providers about any dietary changes you may be considering.

ACUPUNCTURE

Acupuncture is a practice that was developed as a part of traditional Chinese medicine. It involves the stimulation of certain points on the body by a variety of methods, including the insertion and manipulation of thin steel needles or the use of pressure from the practitioner's hands. Some people try acupuncture to treat arthritis pain or inflammation. Reliable research studies have shown that acupuncture can help relieve pain associated with osteoarthritis, but the effect is short-lived. Repeated applications gradually diminish the pain-relieving effect. However, not much is known about acupuncture's effectiveness in treating symptoms of rheumatoid arthritis. A few studies have been conducted, and the findings do not answer this question clearly. Additional, more rigorous research is needed.

Acupuncture tends to have minimal side effects, if any. If you decide to use acupuncture, it is important to find a licensed and certified practitioner, because any complications that have been reported were due to inadequate practitioner training and experience.

REFLEXOLOGY, HOMEOPATHY, THERAPEUTIC TOUCH, NATUROPATHY, AND MAGNETS

Reflexology is the practice of stimulating nerves on the feet and hands in an attempt to favorably influence body functions. Practitioners claim that reflexology reduces stiffness in arthritis; however, there is no research to support that claim.

Homeopathy is an alternative medical practice developed in Germany and brought to the United States in the nineteenth century. It involves administering very small doses of substances called "remedies" that are thought to produce symptoms that are similar to the illness they are being used to treat. This approach is referred to as "like cures like." The remedies are highly diluted. There has been limited research with mixed results on the efficacy of homeopathy in treating arthritis. It appears from some studies that homeopathy might be more effective than a placebo, but this evidence is not strong. More extensive, better-designed studies are needed to resolve this question. Homeopathic remedies are generally considered safe and unlikely to cause severe side effects or interact with conventional drugs.

Proponents of therapeutic touch propose that there are energy fields that go beyond the boundaries of our physical bodies. By entering these energy fields, a practitioner's hands are able to smooth over any problem areas. There is no proof that such energy fields exist.

Naturopathy is a drugless treatment system that employs natural forces such as light, heat, air, water, and massage. The goal of naturopathy is to prevent disease and allow the body to heal itself by natural means. Treatments include nutritional therapy, the use of dietary supplements, promotion of healthy habits, the use of botanical medicines, acupuncture, homeopathy, manipulation, and hypnotherapy. Some of these treatments (discussed previously in this section) are supported by little scientific evidence and should not be used as substitutes for conventional treatment.

**Pregnant women should exercise extreme
caution when it comes to alternative remedies.**

Magnets are objects that produce a type of energy referred to as magnetic fields. The term "magnets" is also used to refer to consumer products that contain magnets. Examples of these include shoe insoles, clothing, wraps for parts of the body, and mattress pads. These products tend to contain so-called static magnets, referred to as such because their magnetic field is unchanging. Research in the use of static magnets does not support claims that they are effective in treating arthritis pain. Magnets can also be very expensive; for example, magnetic insoles may cost $300 or more. Other magnetic devices can cost thousands of dollars and have no proven value. Pregnant women and people who have an acute sprain, an inflammation, an infection, or a wound that can be affected by dilation of the blood vessels should not use static magnets. People who have implanted heart pacemakers and defibrillators (magnets cause malfunction of the device with dire results) and insulin pumps, or who use medication patches, should also avoid magnets altogether.

MIND-BODY TECHNIQUES

Mind-body techniques draw on the interactions that exist in health and disease between the mind, the emotions, the body as a whole, and various body systems, such as the immune, nervous, and endocrine systems. Some mind-body techniques are part of ancient healing traditions; others have emerged in recent times. Examples of mind-body techniques include meditation, tai-chi, relaxation techniques, and spirituality.

Mind-body therapies have been applied to and studied for treating various types of pain. Results of clinical trials indicate that they may be effective additions to the treatment and management of arthritis pain. Studies have noted that mind-body techniques can lead to significant improvements in arthritis pain, disability, overall psychological status, coping ability, and the patient's belief in his or her ability to handle situations (self-efficacy).

There are still questions about mind-body techniques that have not been answered by research, such as which among these therapies are the most effective and, if they work, how they work.

OTHER MISCELLANEOUS CAHC THERAPIES

The list of complimentary and alternative remedies discussed in the previous sections is by no means all-inclusive. Numerous additional remedies have been proposed, but their inclusion here is beyond the scope of this chapter. The list of additional therapies is long and includes copper bracelets, cobra venom, bee-sting therapy, extract of the green-lipped mussel, WD-40, gin-soaked raisins, aromatherapy, polarity therapy, radon pads and uranium mines, rattlesnake meat, ant venom, and so on. They all have been tried with dubious results. It is important to heed the following warning: **If something looks too good to be true, then it probably is.**

Apply the "it-looks-too-good-to-be-true" test to ads for health products by watching for these common warning signs:

✦ A quick and painless cure.

✦ A "special," "secret," "ancient," or "foreign" formula, available only through the mail and only from one supplier.

✦ Personal testimonials or case histories from satisfied users as the only proof that the product works.

✦ A single product that claims to be effective for a variety of ailments.

✦ A scientific "breakthrough" or "miracle cure" that has been held back or overlooked by the medical community.

Consumers in the United States spend more than two billion dollars a year on complimentary and alternative health-care therapies, with very little to show for it. As long as these therapies remain unregulated and unaccountable, they will continue to thrive.

It is no big mystery why patients with arthritis often fall for complimentary and alternative health-care therapies. Western medicine can be impersonal, high-tech, and "cold." Natural medicine is personal, high-touch, and "warm." Western medicine treats you like a collection of organs and parts. Natural medicine treats you like a human being. Even better, a natural healer can see you now, anytime you are in need, and he or she actually has time to talk to you. These healers are not rushing you out the door in 6.5 minutes. They are interested; they care. Not only do they claim to fix your original problem, they also find out what else may be wrong that you are not aware of, and they'll fix that, too. And if you believe in the new treatment enough, it might just work (for a short time anyway). The placebo effect, like the mind-body connection, is a wondrous thing.

So what will work for you? Overall, western medicine is the safest, because it is based on science and good research evidence. But wouldn't it be a wonderful world if conventional health practitioners could learn a few tricks from alternative healers about how to be compassionate and caring and treat the whole person?

Epilogue

We wrote this book to provide you with an in-depth under-standing of how arthritis, a family of relatively common and treatable conditions, can affect you physically and emotionally and to provide you with the key tools you need to manage your arthritis and lead a full and satisfying life. Having arthritis is not easy; pain and physical limitations, are the common denominators in all forms of arthritis–from the benign to the most serious, systemic forms of the disease. But there are positive strategies that you can employ to take control of your health care and stay well in spite of your diagnosis.

Unlike other self-help books on arthritis, our chief focus is not in simply listing the pros and cons of various treatments but rather we strive to provide you with the knowledge and tools you need to make empowered positive decisions for managing your arthritis. The management plan we advocate, one that includes drug therapy, appropriate exercise, pain management, psychosocial support, and other wellness-oriented lifestyle management strategies, has been well tested and delivers good results. The comprehensive treatment recommendations in this book are based on current research findings and the opinions of experts in the field of arthritis. While the medical and surgical therapies covered in this book are commonly used to treat arthritis, the more comprehensive approach to disease management that we advocate here –which includes consideration of all physical and psychosocial factors– is generally underutilized.

We encourage you to do all you can to be well. While staying healthy is a challenge when you have arthritis, you can take steps to live a healthier lifestyle and enjoy real, tangible benefits. The future is brighter than ever before for people with arthritis and the potential for them to live full and productive lives is growing. Ongoing research on this continent, and in other parts of the world, is daily increasing our understanding of this group of diseases and their management. While the search for a cure is intensive, new therapies continue to evolve and offer patients novel and effective treatments.

This section contains information on resources that are helpful to people with arthritis as they learn to manage their condition. As always, when seeking information, keep the following simple rules in mind:

✦ Opt for sources that provide current, well-researched information relative to your type of arthritis. Avoid sources that promise "cures" or "instant relief."

✦ Select information that is easy to access and in language that is simple to understand.

✦ When choosing books or articles, check to see if the author is a recognized expert in the area of interest with good credentials.

✦ Don't hesitate to ask your physician or health care team to evaluate or recommend information and resources.

Organizations

The following not-for-profit organizations are reliable sources of help and information. They typically provide information on types of services and treatments as well as educational materials, publications, and resources and links to support groups for patients and families.

In the United States and Canada

Arthritis Foundation
1330 West Peachtree St. NW
Atlanta, GA 30309
Phone: 1-800-283-7800 (US only)
www.arthritis.org

Lupus Foundation of America Inc.
2000 L Street, N.W., Suite 710
Washington, DC 20036
Phone: 202-349-1155
www.lupus.org

National Fibromyalgia Syndrome Association
2121 S. Towne Centre Place, Suite 300
Anaheim, CA 92806
Phone: 714-921-0150
www.fmaware.org

Spondylitis Association of America
Box 5872
Sherman Oaks, CA 91413
Phone: 1-800-777-8189 (US only)
www.spondylitis.org

The Arthritis Society
393 University Ave. Ste. 1700
Toronto, ON M5G 1E6
Phone: 1-800-321-1433 (Canada only)
www.arthritis.ca

Lupus Canada
590 Alden Road, Suite 211
Markham, ON L3R 8N2
Phone: 1-800-661-1468
www.lupuscanada.org

Outside the United States and Canada

Arthritis Australia
1st floor, 52 Paramatta Road
Forest Lodge, NSW 2037 Australia
Phone: 1-800-111-101 (Australia only)
www.arthritisaustralia.com.au

Arthritis New Zealand
166 Featherston Street
Wellington, New Zealand
Phone 04 472 1427
www.arthritis.org.nz

National Ankylosing Spondylitis Society
BSR
Bride House
18-20 Bride Lane, London EC4Y 8EE
Phone: 44 (0) 20 7842 0900
www.nass.co.uk

Books and Periodicals

There are a host of books available on arthritis and related diseases. Not all books are created equal. When choosing books, consider the authors' credentials and background and beware of sensational claims or promises. The Arthritis Society and the Arthritis Foundation can also recommend a selection of books for you.

Living Well with Arthritis
Authors: Dianne Mosher, Howard Stein, and Gunnar Kraag
Publisher: Penguin Global, 2007

Rheumatoid Arthritis: Plan to Win
Cheryl Koehn, Taysha Palmer, and John Esdaile
Publisher: Oxford University Press, New York, 2002

Arthritis
John Marcus Thompson
Publisher: Key Porter Books, Ontario, Canada, 2005

The Arthritis Helpbook: A Tested Self-Management Program for Coping With Arthritis and Fibromyalgia
(Available in English and French)
Kate Lorig and James Fries
Publisher: Da Capo Books, 2006

The Arthritis Foundation's Tips for Good Living with Arthritis
Shelley Peterman Schwarz with the Arthritis Foundation
Publisher: Arthritis Foundation, 2001

Action Plan for Arthritis
A. Lynn Miller
Publisher: Human Kinetics, 2003

Stop Being Your Symptoms, Start Being Yourself
Arthur Barsky and Emily Deans
Publisher: Harper Collins, 2006

Good Living with Fibromyalgia, Second Edition
Publisher: Arthritis Foundation, 2006

All You Need to Know About Joint Surgery
Publisher: Arthritis Foundation, 2002

Kids Get Arthritis Too—Coloring Book
Publisher: Arthritis Foundation, 1998

Straight Talk on Spondylitis
Publisher: Spondylitis Association of America

Your Child with Arthritis: A Family Guide for Caregiving
Lori Tucker, Bethany DeNardo, Jane Schaller, and Judith Stebulis
Publisher: Johns Hopkins Press, 2000

The Lupus Book
Daniel J. Wallace
Publisher: Oxford University Press, 2005

Periodicals

The following periodicals offer timely information about arthritis and related diseases.

Arthritis Today—bi-monthly magazine available at newstands or through the Arthritis Foundation website, www.arthritis.org.

Lupus Now—magazine published three times per year by the Lupus Foundation of America, available by subscription through their website, www.lupus.org.

Spondylitis Plus—magazine available through membership in the Spondylitis Association of America, www.spondylitis.org.

JointHealth—monthly–newsletter available at www.arthritisconsumerexperts.com.

Audiovisual Materials

Arthritis Foundation
www.arthritis.org
Arthritis Water Exercise – DVD
Take Control with Exercise – DVD and VHS
Walk with Ease—Audiotape

Spondylitis Association of America
www.spondylitis.org
Back in Action—VHS
Exercise Audiotape

Web Sites

Please follow the advice in Chapter 5 regarding the use of the Internet when searching for information and resources. Remember, also that the Internet is an ever-changing entity and addresses often change over time. The Web sites recommended below provide comprehensive and balanced information.

Arthritis Consumer Experts
www.arthritisconsumerexperts.org
Podcasts and a monthly newsletter provide education, advocacy training, and information for people with arthritis.

Healthy Canadians
www.healthycanadians.gc.ca
Easy access to Government of Canada health-related information.

Just for Arthritis Kids
www.arthritiskids.ca
A new interactive Web site for children and parents developed by the Canadian Rheumatology Association and The Arthritis Society.

Cochrane Collaboration
www.cochrane.org
Reliable information for consumers on health care.

Federal Government Programs and Services (Canada)
www.canada.gc.ca

U.S. National Library of Medicine
www.medlineplus/arthritis
Reliable information on a variety of health topics including arthritis.

U.S. Department of Agriculture
www.mypyramid.gov
Information on making smart choices about diet and physical activity.

National Institute of Arthritis and Musculoskeletal and Skin Diseases
National Institutes of Health
www.niams.nih.gov
Information on a wide range of health topics and resources in English and Spanish including access to free publications.

National Psoriasis Foundation/USA
www.psoriasis.org
Disease information, publications, and resources.

Public Health Agency of Canada
www.canadian-health-network.ca
Information on a variety of health and lifestyle topics.

U.S Department of Health and Human Services
www.hhs.gov
Information and links to resources for people with disabilities.

Other Resources

Government Assistance

In some circumstances, government assistance may be available for job retraining, home modifications, disability pensions, and assistive device purchase. Finding these resources is not always easy. Your health care providers may be able to recommend services and programs. Local community health programs can also help you to find the services you need. Another valuable resource is your public library. If you have difficulty searching the Internet, or do not have access to the Internet, the library can assist you with searching for information on government programs, services, and resources in the appropriate jurisdiction– local, state or provincial, or federal.

Assistive Devices

It is wise to consult with your healthcare provider before purchasing any device or aid to assist with your daily activities in order to determine whether or not the device is appropriate and safe. There are many sources for purchasing products of this sort. Devices can be ordered from catalogues, over the Internet, from medical suppliers, pharmacies, or large department stores that often have designated departments for these products. Kitchen and hardware stores can also offer items with larger grips, light-weight tools, and easy-to-use gadgets. Begin your search by checking your yellow pages for local retailers.

Index